Respiratory Disease in the COVID-19 Era

Respiratory Disease in the COVID-19 Era

Editor

Masaki Okamoto

MDPI • Basel • Beijing • Wuhan • Barcelona • Belgrade • Manchester • Tokyo • Cluj • Tianjin

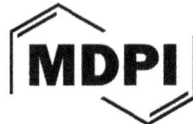

Editor
Masaki Okamoto
Kurume University School of Medicine
Japan

Editorial Office
MDPI
St. Alban-Anlage 66
4052 Basel, Switzerland

This is a reprint of articles from the Special Issue published online in the open access journal *Medicina* (ISSN 1648-9144) (available at: https://www.mdpi.com/journal/medicina/special_issues/Pulmonary_Fibrosis_COVID).

For citation purposes, cite each article independently as indicated on the article page online and as indicated below:

LastName, A.A.; LastName, B.B.; LastName, C.C. Article Title. *Journal Name* **Year**, *Volume Number*, Page Range.

ISBN 978-3-0365-7916-0 (Hbk)
ISBN 978-3-0365-7917-7 (PDF)

© 2023 by the authors. Articles in this book are Open Access and distributed under the Creative Commons Attribution (CC BY) license, which allows users to download, copy and build upon published articles, as long as the author and publisher are properly credited, which ensures maximum dissemination and a wider impact of our publications.

The book as a whole is distributed by MDPI under the terms and conditions of the Creative Commons license CC BY-NC-ND.

Contents

About the Editor . . . . **vii**

Masaki Okamoto
Special Issue: "Respiratory Disease in the COVID-19 Era"
Reprinted from: *Medicina* 2023, *59*, 886, doi:10.3390/medicina59050886 . . . . **1**

**María Fernanda del Valle, Jorge Valenzuela, Gabriel Nasri Marzuca-Nassr,
Consuelo Cabrera-Inostroza, Mariano del Sol, Pablo A. Lizana, et al.**
Eight Weeks of Supervised Pulmonary Rehabilitation Are Effective in Improving Resting Heart
Rate and Heart Rate Recovery in Severe COVID-19 Patient Survivors of Mechanical Ventilation
Reprinted from: *Medicina* 2022, *58*, 514, doi:10.3390/medicina58040514 . . . . **3**

**Efrén Murillo-Zamora, Xóchitl Trujillo, Miguel Huerta, Mónica Riós-Silva,
José Guzmán-Esquivel, Jaime Alberto Bricio-Barrios, et al.**
COVID-19 Pneumonia in Fully Vaccinated Adults during the Dominance of the Omicron
Sublineages BA.1.1 and BA.2 in Mexico
Reprinted from: *Medicina* 2022, *58*, 1127, doi:10.3390/medicina58081127 . . . . **17**

**Tomoyuki Takahashi, Atsushi Saito, Koji Kuronuma, Hirotaka Nishikiori and
Hirofumi Chiba**
Pneumocystis jirovecii Pneumonia Associated with COVID-19 in Patients with Interstitial
Pneumonia
Reprinted from: *Medicina* 2022, *58*, 1151, doi:10.3390/medicina58091151 . . . . **23**

**Camelia Corina Pescaru, Monica Steluța Marc, Emanuela Oana Costin, Andrei Pescaru,
Ana-Adriana Trusculescu, Adelina Maritescu, et al.**
Massive Spontaneous Pneumomediastinum—A Form of Presentation for Severe COVID-19
Pneumonia
Reprinted from: *Medicina* 2022, *58*, 1525, doi:10.3390/medicina58111525 . . . . **29**

**Tamara Mirela Porosnicu, Ciprian Gindac, Sonia Popovici, Adelina Marinescu, Daniel Jipa,
Valentina Lazaroiu, et al.**
Efficacy of Therapeutic Plasma Exchange in Severe Acute Respiratory Distress Syndrome in
COVID-19 Patients from the Western Part of Romania
Reprinted from: *Medicina* 2022, *58*, 1707, doi:10.3390/medicina58121707 . . . . **35**

**Yoji Nagasaki, Masanori Kadowaki, Asako Nakamura, Yoshiki Etoh, Masatoshi Shimo,
Sayoko Ishihara, et al.**
A Case of a Malignant Lymphoma Patient Persistently Infected with SARS-CoV-2 for More than
6 Months
Reprinted from: *Medicina* 2023, *59*, 108, doi:10.3390/medicina59010108 . . . . **45**

**Jun Sasaki, Masanobu Matsuoka, Takashi Kinoshita, Takayuki Horii, Shingo Tsuneyoshi,
Daiki Murata, et al.**
A Cluster of Paragonimiasis with Delayed Diagnosis Due to Difficulty Distinguishing
Symptoms from Post-COVID-19 Respiratory Symptoms: A Report of Five Cases
Reprinted from: *Medicina* 2023, *59*, 137, doi:10.3390/medicina59010137 . . . . **53**

**Sebastiano Cicco, Marialuisa Sveva Marozzi, Carmen Alessandra Palumbo,
Elisabetta Sturdà, Antonio Fusillo, Flavio Scarilli, et al.**
Lung Ultrasound Is Useful for Evaluating Lung Damage in COVID-19 Patients Treated with
Bamlanivimab and Etesevimab: A Single-Center Pilot Study
Reprinted from: *Medicina* 2023, *59*, 203, doi:10.3390/medicina59020203 . . . . **59**

Muiez Bashir, Wani Inzamam, Irfan Robbani, Tanveer Rasool Banday, Fahad A. Al-Misned, Hamed A. El-Serehy and Carmen Vladulescu
Patients with Diabetes Experienced More Serious and Protracted Sickness from the COVID-19 Infection: A Prospective Study
Reprinted from: *Medicina* **2023**, *59*, 472, doi:10.3390/medicina59030472 71

Tomohiro Tanaka, Masaki Okamoto, Norikazu Matsuo, Yoshiko Naitou-Nishida, Takashi Nouno, Takashi Kojima, et al.
Case Series of Patients with Coronavirus Disease 2019 Pneumonia Treated with Hydroxychloroquine
Reprinted from: *Medicina* **2023**, *59*, 541, doi:10.3390/medicina59030541 83

Yang-Jin Lee
Thoracic Mobilization and Respiratory Muscle Endurance Training Improve Diaphragm Thickness and Respiratory Function in Patients with a History of COVID-19
Reprinted from: *Medicina* **2023**, *59*, 906, doi:10.3390/medicina59050906 93

About the Editor

Masaki Okamoto

Masaki Okamoto, M.D. and Ph.D. I am an associate professor at the Department of Respirology, National Hospital Organization Kyushu Medical Center, and Chief Doctor of the Division of Respirology, Neurology, and Rheumatology, Kurume University. My study field is respirology, particularly diffuse lung disease.

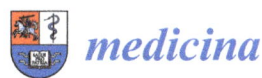

Editorial

Special Issue: "Respiratory Disease in the COVID-19 Era"

Masaki Okamoto

Department of Respirology and Clinical Research Center, National Hospital Organization Kyushu Medical Center, 1-8-1 Jigyohama, Chuo-ku, Fukuoka 810-0065, Japan; okamoto_masaki@med.kurume-u.ac.jp; Tel.: +81-92-852-0700; Fax: +81-92-847-8802

The outbreak of the viral infection known as coronavirus disease 2019 (COVID-19), caused by the novel pathogen severe acute respiratory syndrome coronavirus-2 (SARS-CoV-2), was first reported in Wuhan, China, in December 2019. Thereafter, the illness spread rapidly across the world [1]. The development of acute respiratory distress syndrome has remained the most significant risk factor for acute COVID-19-related mortality since the beginning of the outbreak [1–3]. In a study by Wu et al., 44 (52.4%) of 84 patients who developed acute respiratory distress syndrome attributable to COVID-19 died^2. Aggravating factors for this condition include older age, obesity with diabetes mellitus as a complication, hypertension, and malignant disease [2,3].

COVID-19-related pneumonia exhibits specific radiological features upon high-resolution computed tomography. Li et al. found that patients with COVID-19-related pneumonia were more likely to have rounded opacities (35% vs. 17%) and interlobular septal thickening (66% vs. 43%), and were less likely to have nodules (28% vs. 71%), the tree-in-bud sign (9% vs. 40%), or pleural effusion (6% vs. 31%), when compared with patients who had influenza-related pneumonia [4].

Randomized controlled trials and observational studies of various immunosuppressive therapies have been performed in patients with COVID-19-related pneumonia. A meta-analysis suggested that corticosteroid therapy resulted in delayed virus clearance and did not improve survival or decrease the length hospital stays, the rate of admission to intensive care units, and/or the use of mechanical ventilation in patients with SARS-CoV-2, SARS-CoV, or MERS-CoV infection [5]. However, some studies have found no difference in the time to clearance of SARS-CoV-2 RNA regardless of whether corticosteroid therapy is administered [6]. The controlled open-label RECOVERY trial compared mortality between patients with COVID-19 who received oral or intravenous dexamethasone at a dosage of 6 mg, once daily, for up to 10 days and those who received standard care alone. The 28-day mortality rate (i.e., the primary outcome) was lower in patients with moderate or severe COVID-19 who received dexamethasone than in those who received standard care [7]. However, no benefit was seen in patients with mild COVID-19. In a prospective meta-analysis of 10,930 patients with COVID-19 that compared the outcomes of patients who received standard care with those of patients who received a placebo, the administration of tocilizumab and interleukin-6 antagonists was associated with lower 28-day all-cause mortality [8]. To date, the only drugs that show evidence of reducing mortality in patients with COVID-19 are corticosteroids. This finding contrasts with the results of a meta-analysis showing that corticosteroid therapy increases mortality in patients with influenza [9].

One of the chronic sequelae of COVID-19 is residual respiratory impairment after acute pneumonia. A systematic review of 13 studies that included a total of 2018 patients found that about 44.9% of COVID-19 survivors developed pulmonary fibrosis [10].

The spread of COVID-19 is abating, but is not converging. Therefore, this Special Issue presents basic and clinical research on this disease.

Acknowledgments: We thank all collaborators.

Conflicts of Interest: The author declares no conflict of interest.

References

1. Huang, C.; Wang, Y.; Li, X.; Ren, L.; Zhao, J.; Hu, Y.; Zhang, L.; Fan, G.; Xu, J.; Gu, X.; et al. Clinical features of patients infected with 2019 novel coronavirus in Wuhan, China. *Lancet* **2020**, *395*, 497–506. [CrossRef] [PubMed]
2. Wu, C.; Chen, X.; Cai, Y.; Zhou, X.; Xu, S.; Huang, H.; Zhang, L.; Zhou, X.; Du, C.; Zhang, Y.; et al. Risk factors associated with acute respiratory distress syndrome and death in patients with coronavirus disease 2019 pneumonia in Wuhan, China. *JAMA Intern. Med.* **2020**, *180*, 934–943. [CrossRef] [PubMed]
3. Wang, D.; Hu, B.; Hu, C.; Zhu, F.; Liu, X.; Zhang, J.; Wang, B.; Xiang, H.; Cheng, Z.; Xiong, Y.; et al. Clinical characteristics of 138 hospitalized patients with 2019 novel coronavirus-infected pneumonia in Wuhan, China. *JAMA* **2020**, *323*, 1061–1069. [CrossRef] [PubMed]
4. Liu, M.; Zeng, W.; Wen, Y.; Zheng, Y.; Lv, F.; Xiao, K. COVID-19 pneumonia: CT findings of 122 patients and differentiation from influenza pneumonia. *Eur. Radiol.* **2020**, *30*, 5463–5469. [CrossRef] [PubMed]
5. Li, H.; Chen, C.; Hu, F.; Wang, J.; Zhao, Q.; Gale, R.P.; Liang, Y. Impact of corticosteroid therapy on outcomes of persons with SARS-CoV-2, SARS-CoV, or MERS-CoV infection: A systematic review and meta-analysis. *Leukemia* **2020**, *34*, 1503–1511. [CrossRef] [PubMed]
6. Fang, X.; Mei, Q.; Yang, T.; Li, L.; Wang, Y.; Tong, F.; Geng, S.; Pan, A. Low-dose corticosteroid therapy does not delay viral clearance in patients with COVID-19. *J. Infect.* **2020**, *81*, 147–178. [CrossRef] [PubMed]
7. Recovery Collaborative Group. Dexamethasone in hospitalized patients with COVID-19. *N. Engl. J. Med.* **2021**, *384*, 693–704. [CrossRef] [PubMed]
8. Domingo, P.; Mur, I.; Mateo, G.M.; del Mar Gutierrez, M.; Pomar, V.; de Benito, N.; Corbacho, N.; Herrera, S.; Millan, L.; Muñoz, J.; et al. Association between administration of IL-6 antagonists and mortality among patients hospitalized for COVID-19: A meta-analysis. *JAMA* **2021**, *326*, 499–518.
9. Lansbury, L.E.; Rodrigo, C.; Leonardi-Bee, J.; Nguyen-Van-Tam, J.; Shen Lim, W. Corticosteroids as adjunctive therapy in the treatment of influenza: An updated Cochrane systematic review and meta-analysis. *Crit. Care Med.* **2020**, *48*, e98–e106. [CrossRef]
10. Amin, B.J.H.; Kakamad, F.H.; Ahmed, G.S.; Ahmed, S.F.; Abdulla, B.A.; Mikael, T.M.; Salih, R.Q.; Salh, A.M.; Hussein, D.A. Post COVID-19 pulmonary fibrosis: A meta-analysis study. *Ann. Med. Surg.* **2022**, *77*, 103590.

Disclaimer/Publisher's Note: The statements, opinions and data contained in all publications are solely those of the individual author(s) and contributor(s) and not of MDPI and/or the editor(s). MDPI and/or the editor(s) disclaim responsibility for any injury to people or property resulting from any ideas, methods, instructions or products referred to in the content.

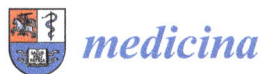

Article

Eight Weeks of Supervised Pulmonary Rehabilitation Are Effective in Improving Resting Heart Rate and Heart Rate Recovery in Severe COVID-19 Patient Survivors of Mechanical Ventilation

María Fernanda del Valle [1], Jorge Valenzuela [1], Gabriel Nasri Marzuca-Nassr [2], Consuelo Cabrera-Inostroza [1], Mariano del Sol [3], Pablo A. Lizana [4], Máximo Escobar-Cabello [5] and Rodrigo Muñoz-Cofre [1,6,*]

1. Servicio de Medicina Física y Rehabilitación, Hospital el Carmen, Maipú 9251521, Chile; fer.delvalle91@gmail.com (M.F.d.V.); jorge.valenzuelav@redsalud.gob.cl (J.V.); consuelocabrera@hotmail.com (C.C.-I.)
2. Departamento de Medicina Interna, Facultad de Medicina, Universidad de La Frontera, Temuco 4781218, Chile; gabriel.marzuca@ufrontera.cl
3. Centro de Excelencia en Estudios Morfológicos y Quirúrgicos, Universidad de La Frontera, Temuco 4811230, Chile; mariano.delsol@ufrontera.cl
4. Laboratory of Epidemiology and Morphological Sciences, Instituto de Biología, Pontificia Universidad Católica de Valparaíso, Valparaíso 2373223, Chile; pablo.lizana@pucv.cl
5. Laboratorio de Función Disfunción Ventilatoria, Departamento de Kinesiología, Universidad Católica del Maule, Talca 3480112, Chile; maxfescobar@gmail.com
6. Posdoctorado en Ciencias Morfológicas, Universidad de La Frontera, Temuco 4811230, Chile
* Correspondence: rodrigomunozcofre@gmail.com; Tel.: +56-97-8970-129

Abstract: *Background and Objectives*: Patients who survive severe COVID-19 require significant pulmonary rehabilitation. Heart rate (HR) has been used as a safety variable in the evaluation of the results of interventions in patients undergoing pulmonary rehabilitation. The aim of this research was to analyse HR during a pulmonary rehabilitation program in post-severe COVID-19 patients who survived mechanical ventilation (MV). The study includes the initial and final evaluations and aerobic training sessions. *Materials and Methods:* Twenty patients (58 ± 13 years, 11 men) were trained for 8 weeks. A 6-minute walk test (6 MWT) was performed and, subsequently, a supervised and individualised training plan was created. Resting heart rate (RHR), heart rate recovery (HRR), heart rate at minute 6 (HR6 min) and the product of HR6 min and systolic blood pressure (HR6 min$^{\times}$SBP) were measured at 6 MWT. In addition, HR was measured at each training session. *Results:* After 8 weeks of pulmonary rehabilitation, patients decreased their RHR from 81.95 ± 9.36 to 73.60 ± 9.82 beats/min ($p < 0.001$) and significantly increased their HRR from 12.45 ± 10.22 to 20.55 ± 7.33 beats/min ($p = 0.005$). HR6 min presented a significant relationship with walking speed and walked distance after the pulmonary rehabilitation period ($r = 0.555$, $p = 0.011$ and $r = 0.613$, $p = 0.011$, respectively). HR6 min$^{\times}$SBP presented a significant relationship with walking speed and walked distance after training ($r = 0.538$, $p = 0.014$ and $r = 0.568$, $p = 0.008$, respectively). In the pulmonary rehabilitation sessions, a significant decrease in HR was observed at minutes 1, 6 and 15 ($p < 0.05$) between sessions 1 and 6 and at minute 1 between sessions 1 and 12. *Conclusions:* Eight weeks of individualised and supervised pulmonary rehabilitation were effective in improving RHR and HRR in COVID-19 patients surviving MV. HR is an easily accessible indicator that could help to monitor the evaluation and development of a pulmonary rehabilitation program in COVID-19 patients who survived MV.

Keywords: heart rate; COVID-19; pulmonary rehabilitation

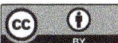

1. Introduction

COVID-19 is a disease caused by the SARS-CoV-2 virus, belonging to the coronavirus family [1]. In December 2019, the World Health Organization (WHO) in China warned about patients with pneumonia of an unknown aetiology and the first case in Chile was registered on 3 March 2020 [1,2]. This marked the beginning of a pandemic that has since affected the entire world [3]. The projections of the functional consequences of this syndemic are still a matter of speculation [4].

Due to severe respiratory symptoms and, in some cases, acute respiratory distress, patients with COVID-19 may require prolonged mechanical ventilation (MV). In addition to MV being an invasive procedure, there are cases where its disconnection can take time. The consequences of prolonged connection to MV generate the need for pulmonary rehabilitation during and after hospitalization [5]. These MV-related complications can include respiratory problems, cognitive problems, myopathies, neuropathies, joint pain, muscle pain, physical deconditioning and cardiac disorders [4–6]. In this sense, the American Thoracic Society-European Respiratory Society (ATS-ERS) suggests that aerobic exercise should be part of a pulmonary rehabilitation program. However, this should be structured individually, after a formal evaluation, due to the cardiorespiratory sequelae caused by COVID-19 [7]. Therefore, heart rate (HR) control in the training evaluation and implementation process would be useful [8], considering the linear relationship between oxygen uptake and cardiac output or HR during functional tests [9].

Some symptoms of COVID-19 can last beyond the period of acute infection, with exercise intolerance standing out as the most frequent finding [7,8,10]. This can occur together with chest pain, dyspnoea, palpitations or even postural orthostatic tachycardia [7]. Exercise intolerance can cause a limitation of activities, resulting in an effort that goes beyond daily life or inactivity [7,8]. Here, the restriction of movement becomes a confounding factor instead of a protective factor [9]. Therefore, the monitoring of HR upon return to exercise is recommended, with the purpose of observing the exercise behaviour of patients who survived COVID-19 [8] and also to determine whether there is an indirect impact of pulmonary rehabilitation on the cardiopulmonary system.

Baseline fitness assessment through the 6-minute walk test (6 MWT) and aerobic training are part of most pulmonary rehabilitation programs [7,11]. Thus, changes in HR with various interventions that increase physical workload may be useful in assessing an exercise training risk profile [8,11]. It has been reported that the decrease in HR at rest related to physical activity decreases the incidence of cardiovascular diseases, in addition to having a positive impact on all-cause mortality [12,13]. On the other hand, heart rate recovery (HRR) shows autonomic activity in the cardiovascular system and has also been shown to be a predictor of morbidity and mortality in patients with heart failure [14]. In this context, the aim of this study was to analyse HR during a pulmonary rehabilitation program in post-severe COVID-19 patients who survived MV, including the initial and final evaluations and aerobic training sessions. In this sense, our research hypothesis is that the intervention, through an 8-week pulmonary rehabilitation program, would decrease resting heart rate (RHR) and improve HRR.

2. Materials and Methods

2.1. Participants

This was a prospective study, where the sample was for convenience and the recruitment of participants to the pulmonary rehabilitation program was in accordance with bronchopulmonary dysplasia. Twenty patients (58 ± 13 years old; 11 men and 9 women) diagnosed with COVID-19 were included in the present study. This research was approved by the Scientific Ethics Committee of the Central Metropolitan Health Service (Resolution No. 048975). In addition, all patients read and signed an informed consent agreement. The inclusion criteria were as follows: (a) diagnosis of severe/critical COVID-19, (b) requirement of MV with orotracheal intubation, (c) hospital discharge, (d) control with a cardiologist and normal electrocardiogram and (e) being in health control at the Carmen

Hospital in Maipú, Santiago, Chile. Patients who did not understand commands were excluded. All participants underwent 8 weeks of individualised and supervised pulmonary rehabilitation. In these 8 weeks, 2 evaluation sessions (PRE and POST), 12 exercise sessions and 2 control sessions (after completion of pulmonary rehabilitation) were included. Before (PRE) and after (POST) pulmonary rehabilitation, the walked distance with the 6 MWT was evaluated, and the RHR, HRR, heart rate at minute 6 (HR6 min) and product of the HR6 min with systolic blood pressure (SBP) (HR6 min$^\times$SBP) were measured in this test. Ventilatory capacity through spirometry was also performed before and after 8 weeks of pulmonary rehabilitation. In addition, an incremental and continuous test was carried out to design the pulmonary rehabilitation sessions. HR was also measured at each training session.

2.2. Test Day

The test period consisted of two identical evaluation days before and after the pulmonary rehabilitation period. The participants arrived at the hospital and underwent an evaluation of their baseline parameters (blood pressure, HR, weight and height) and then performed a spirometry test. After a 10-minute rest, a 6 MWT was performed with the measurement of the parameters indicated above before and after the test. The 6 MWT was used to measure the walked distance by each participant and their walking speed, which allowed the incremental test to be dosed according to the conditions of each participant. The continuous test was used to evaluate the duration of the maximum speed obtained in the incremental test. The three tests (6 MWT, continuous test and incremental test) were performed on the same day, with 10 min of rest between each one and always in the same order.

2.2.1. Spirometry

Spirometric measurements were standardised according to the standards of the American Thoracic Society [15], incorporating national suggestions in relation to care due to the COVID-19 pandemic [16]. The patient, in a seated position, placed the pneumotachograph in his/her mouth and forced expiration was requested based on total lung capacity. The values of forced vital capacity (FVC), which is the volume that has been exhaled at the end of the first second of forced expiration (FEV1), and their ratio (FEV1/FVC) were considered. For this, a Medgraphics spirometer (CPFS/D USB 2.02, MGC Diagnostics Corporation, Saint Paul, MN, USA) was used [17].

2.2.2. Walked Distance and Heart Rate Parameters

In this study, 6 MWT was held in a 30-metre-long corridor, free of traffic. According to Muñoz et al., with constant stimulation, patients were instructed to walk as many metres as possible during the corresponding six minutes [18]. Dyspnoea and lower limb fatigue were categorised using the modified Borg scale [19]. Oximetry was measured at the beginning and end of the test by a pulse oximeter (Nonin 7500®, Nonin Medical, Minneapolis, MN, USA). The walked distance was recorded in metres. HR was recorded using the Polar® system (Polar® FT2, Kempele, Finland). An elastic belt (Polar T31 transmitter, Polar Electro, Kempele, Finland) was attached to the participant's chest at the level of the lower third of the sternum. In the 6 MWT, HR was recorded at rest, during the 6 MWT and in the recovery period (one minute after completion of the 6 MWT) [18,20]. The HRs used were the following: (1) HRH, (2) heart rate at minute 6 (HR6 min) [9], (3) HRR = HR at minute 6 of the 6 MWT minus the HR at one minute after the completion of the 6 MWT [20] and (4) the product of HR6 min and systolic pressure at minute 6 of 6 MWT (HR6 min$^\times$SBP) [13]. In addition, HR was measured in each pulmonary rehabilitation session; at minutes 1, 3, 6, 10, 15, 20, 25 and 30; and in recovery (1 and 5 min).

2.2.3. Incremental Test

The incremental test was performed on a treadmill (Spirit CT800 212089®, Jonesboro, AR, USA). The loads used in each stage of the incremental test were calculated from the average speed obtained in the 6 MWT, with the method described above [21]. Using a known distance and a stopwatch, the time it took for the patient to travel 30 m was measured. Gait speed was calculated using the following equation: speed = distance/time (m/sec). Subsequently, the conversion was made to km/h, a unit to be programmed in the treadmill. The maximum speed or 100% was the average obtained from each turn. The initial stage was using 45% speed on the 6 MWT and an incline of 1. The speed was in-creased by 15% and the incline level was also increased every 1 min. Once 100% of the speed calculated through the 6 MWT was reached and in the absence of test suspension criteria, the speed continued to increase by 15% every minute [22]. HR, dyspnoea and fatigue were assessed at each minute of the session. The test was stopped when the patient presented dyspnoea or fatigue $\geq$ 7 points, a pulse saturometry of <91% and/or exceeded 80% of their heart rate reserve [23].

2.2.4. Continuous Test

This procedure was performed on the same treadmill described above at constant speed, using the stage immediately prior to stopping the incremental test [24]. The test was stopped when the participant presented dyspnoea or fatigue $\geq$ 7 points, a pulse saturometry of <91% and/or exceeded 80% of their heart rate reserve [22]. The information obtained in this test made it possible to determine whether the participant was able to tolerate the load proposed for interval training. Both in the incremental test and the continuous test, the measurements associated with dyspnoea and fatigue were made using a visual analogue scale, according to the Borg scale [19].

3. Pulmonary Rehabilitation Program

The exercise sessions were carried out twice a week in person for two months (November 2020 to January 2021). Each face-to-face session was divided into 30 min of aerobic training, 20 min of strength training and 10 min of flexibility training. The sessions were individual, directed and supervised by a physical therapist. In addition, the inspiratory muscle strength training was performed by the patient at home under the indication of the physical therapist. Workloads in aerobic exercise were performed with the results of the previously described incremental and continuous tests.

3.1. Face-To-Face Sessions

3.1.1. Aerobic Training

Prior to each session, bronchodilation was performed with 200 mcg of salbutamol, because no patient had saturation problems or was an oxygen user. Oxygen was only used in aerobic training; it was supported with two litres of oxygen through the nose or according to the pulse oximetry of each patient in exercise. Aerobic training was performed on a treadmill. The work strategy used was interval training, where 60% and 80% of the speed and inclination obtained in the incremental test were maintained for two and three minutes, respectively [22]. The criteria for stopping the training session were the same used in the incremental and continuous tests, in addition to the symptoms of inadequacy to exercise such as dizziness, headache and pain. Aerobic workloads were used from the values obtained in the incremental and continuous tests (Table 1).

3.1.2. Strength Training

In the first instance, a warm-up and joint mobility of the whole body were performed, after which lower limb exercises were performed using semi-squats and medium-resistance elastic bands (green; Theraband, Hygenic Co., Akron, OH, USA), and finally, muscle chain exercises were performed bilaterally (biceps, triceps, trapezius, latissimus dorsi, abdominals and hip abductors). An exercise progression sequence was followed, starting with two sets of 10 repetitions, with 20 s of rest between each series, to conclude the intervention with three sets of 25 repetitions and 20 s of rest between each series (Table 1) [25].

Table 1. Description of the pulmonary rehabilitation program.

	Face-to-Face Sessions (2×/week)					Home Sessions (Every Day)
Aerobic Training	Strength Training				Flexibility Training	Inspiratory Muscle Training
	Upper-body	Set/Rep.	Lower-body	Set/Rep.		
30 min of walking on a treadmill.	Bilateral muscle chain exercises of: Biceps	2/10 3/25	Half squats.	2/10 3/25	Two series of 15 seconds for biceps, triceps, trapezius, and latissimus dorsi.	Twice a day: Between 7:00 a.m.–12:00 a.m.: 30 % MIP 3 series of 3 minutes with 2 minutes of rest.
Interval work: 2 min at 60% speed and incline obtained in the incremental test. 3 min at 80% speed and incline obtained in the incremental test	Triceps	2/10 3/25	Hip abductors with medium resistance elastic bands	2/10 3/25	Two series of 15 seconds for quadriceps, hamstrings, and triceps surae.	Between 4:00 p.m.–9:00 p.m.: 30 % MIP 3 series of 3 minutes with 2 minutes of rest.
	Trapezius	2/10 3/25				
	Latissimus dorsi	2/10 3/25				

Rep: repetitions; MIP: maximum inspiratory pressure.

3.1.3. Flexibility Training

Each session ended with flexibility exercises that consisted of muscle stretching for each muscle group worked (2 series × 15 s of maintenance), concentrating on the inhalation and exhalation process [26]. If the patient reported joint pain after the training session, cryotherapy was used for 20 min (Table 1) [27].

3.2. At Home Sessions
Inspiratory Muscle Training

This was performed at home with a threshold valve (Philips Respironics, NJ, USA) IMT (Inspiratory Muscle Trainer), twice a day (morning: between 7:00 a.m. and 12:00 p.m.; afternoon: between 4:00 p.m. and 9:00 p.m.), for each day of the eight-week pulmonary rehabilitation program. The threshold valve was set at 30% of the initial maximum inspiratory pressure (MIP). The established training protocol consisted of three series of 3 min of training with 2 min of rest; breaths should be slow and deep. The evaluation and progression of the training had to be recorded in a daily record guideline, which was evaluated by the physical therapists in charge of each face-to-face session. Training load was readjusted weekly and MIP was reassessed at the end of the program (Table 1) [28].

4. Safety

Work was carried out in a 24 m^2 box with an exhaust fan, under the care standards implemented by the de Hospital El Carmen in Maipú, Santiago, Chile, during the pandemic, where only the kinesiologist and the patient were present. Rotation was every 60 min and all instruments were cleaned with 70% isopropyl alcohol. The kinesiologist used an N95 mask and face shield and the patient used an N95 mask (3M, St. Paul, MN, USA).

5. Statistical Analysis

The results are presented as means, standard deviation and 95% confidence intervals. The statistical program used was STATA 16 (StataCorp. Stata Statistical Software, College Station, TX, USA). The normality of data was determined through the Shapiro–Wilk test. For the statistical analysis of HR in the 6 MWT, the Student *t*-test or Wilcoxon test for paired samples was used. For the analysis of HR between training sessions, ANOVA was used for repeated measures. For the analysis of dyspnoea and fatigue data, the Friedman test was used. Correlations were established using the Pearson or Spearman coefficient, depending on the normality of the data. A significance level of $p < 0.05$ was considered.

6. Results

6.1. Anthropometry and Spirometry

Twenty-two patients were trained, but two did not complete the eight-week intervention due to voluntary withdrawal, so the results of 20 patients (11 men and 9 women) were analysed. The baseline anthropometric and lung function characteristics of the patients evaluated are shown in Table 2. Weight, body mass index (BMI) and FVC significantly increased after the pulmonary rehabilitation program (Table 3).

Table 2. Baseline characteristics of the participants.

Variable	Mean ± SD
Age (years)	58 ± 13
Weight (kg)	81.69 ± 15.32
Height (cm)	163.4 ± 8.63
BMI (kg/m^2)	30.53 ± 4.56
Obesity (n/%)	11/55
Diabetes Mellitus (n/%)	11/55
Hypertension (n/%)	13/65
Smoking habit (n/%)	0/0
Length of MV (days)	26.82 ± 14.14
Length of ICU (days)	31.03 ± 15.22
Length of hospitalization (days)	39.94 ± 17.74
Time to enter the program (days)	62.47 ± 30.08

BMI: body mass index; MV: mechanical ventilation; n: number; %: percentage; SD: standard deviation; ICU: intensive care unit.

Table 3. Spirometric characteristics in COVID-19 participants before and after a pulmonary rehabilitation program.

	PRE	POST	p Value
FVC (L)	3.17 ± 0.97	3.30 ± 0.94	0.001 ^{w}
FVC pred (%)	86.95 ± 18.94	90.40 ± 16.71	0.001 ^{t}
FEV$_1$ (L)	2.671 ± 0.84	2.71 ± 0.84	0.558 ^{w}
FEV$_1$ pred (%)	89.71 ± 25.18	92.95 ± 16.38	0.269 ^{w}
FEV$_1$/FVC	85.05 ± 5.03	84.25 ± 5.26	0.250 ^{t}

PRE: before starting the pulmonary rehabilitation program; POST: after the pulmonary rehabilitation program; FVC: forced vital capacity; FEV$_1$: volume that has been exhaled at the end of the first second of forced expiration; L: litres; ^{t}: Student t-test; ^{w}: Wilcoxon test.

6.2. Heart Rate and 6-Minute Walk Test Performance

RHR significantly decreased from 81.95 ± 9.36 (95% CI: 77.57–86.33) to 73.60 ± 9.82 (95% CI: 69.00–78.20) beats/min ($p = 0.0008$). HRR increased significantly from 12.45 ± 10.22 (95% CI: 7.66–17.23) to 20.55 ± 7.33 beats/min (95% CI: 17.12–23.98) ($p = 0.005$). HR6 min and HR6 min$^\times$ SBP did not show significant differences after the pulmonary rehabilitation program ($p > 0.05$). Both walking speed and walked distance in the 6 MWT increased significantly from 4.70 ± 1.15 (95% CI: 3.98–5.41) to 5.73 ± 0.99 km/h (95% CI: 5.26–6.19) ($p < 0.001$) and from 451.5 ± 152.2 (95% CI: 380.2–522.7) to 549.3 ± 83.04 (95% CI: 510.4–588.1) metres ($p < 0.001$), respectively (Table 4).

Table 4. Heart rate, perception and performance of the 6 MWT before and after a pulmonary rehabilitation program.

	PRE		POST		
	Mean ± DS	CI 95%	Mean ± DS	CI 95%	p Value
RHR (bpm)	81.95 ± 9.36	(77.57–86.33)	73.60 ± 9.82	(69.00–78.20)	<0.001 ^{t}
HR6 min (bpm)	104.6 ± 16.88	(96.65–112.)	107.6 ± 18.50	(98.94–116.3)	0.381 ^{t}
HRR (bpm)	12.45 ± 10.22	(7.66–17.23)	20.55 ± 7.33	(17.12–23.98)	0.005 ^{t}
HR6 min×SBP	15,715 ± 3021	(14,301–17,129)	14,978 ± 3338	(13,416–16,541)	0.218 ^{t}
Dyspnoea (points)	3 (1–7)	(2.28–3.71)	3 (0–7)	(1.57–3.52)	0.376 ^{w}
Fatigue (points)	3 (0–6)	(2.08–3.91)	2 (0–8)	(1.56–3.73)	0.658 ^{w}
Velocity (km/h)	4.70 ± 1.15	(3.98–5.41)	5.73 ± 0.99	(5.26–6.19)	<0.001 ^{w}
Walked distance (m)	451.5 ± 152.2	(380.2–522.7)	549.3 ± 83.04	(510.4–588.1)	<0.001 ^{w}

The variables are expressed as mean ± standard deviation, dyspnoea and fatigue are expressed as median (minimum–maximum). PRE: before starting the pulmonary rehabilitation program; POST: after the pulmonary rehabilitation program; RHR: resting heart rate; HR6 min: heart rate at minute 6; HRR: heart rate recovery; bpm: beats per minute; SBP: systolic blood pressure; CI: confidence interval; SD: standard deviation; ^{t}: Student t-test; ^{w}: Wilcoxon test.

6.3. Control Parameters between Pulmonary Rehabilitation Sessions

Between sessions 1 and 6 of the pulmonary rehabilitation program, a significant decrease in HR was observed at minutes 1, 6 and 15. In addition, a significant decrease in HR was observed between sessions 1 and 12 at minute 1. The walking speed in each session increased significantly from session 1 to 6 ($p = 0.040$) and from session 1 to 12 ($p < 0.05$) (Figure 1A,C). Similarly, the incline increased significantly from sessions 1 to 6 ($p < 0.05$) and from sessions 1 to 12 ($p < 0.05$) (Figure 1A,C). The subjective sensation of dyspnoea decreased significantly between sessions 1 and 6 at minutes 6, 10, 15, 20, 25 and 30 and between sessions 1 and 12 at minutes 10, 15, 20, 25 and 30 (Figure 2B). The subjective feeling of fatigue decreased significantly between sessions 1 and 6 at minutes 10, 20, 25 and 30 and between sessions 1 and 12 at minutes 10, 15, 20, 25 and 30 (Figure 2C).

6.4. Relationship of the Products of Heart Rate with Speed and Walked Distance in the 6-Min Walk Tests

HR6 min showed significant relationships before and after the pulmonary rehabilitation program. The relationships with speed and walked distance prior to the pulmonary rehabilitation program were r = 0.535, $p = 0.015$ and r = 0.528, $p = 0.016$, respectively. After the pulmonary rehabilitation program, the relationships of HR6 min with speed and walked distance were r = 0.555, $p = 0.011$ and r = 0.613, $p = 0.011$, respectively (Table 5). The HRR with the speed and distance walked before the pulmonary rehabilitation program did not show any significant relationships. However, after pulmonary rehabilitation, HRR had a significant relationship with walked distance (r = 0.461; $p = 0.040$) (Table 5). The HR6 min×SBP, both before and after the pulmonary rehabilitation program, showed significant correlations with walking speed (PRE: r = 0.457, $p = 0.042$ and POST: r = 0.538, $p = 0.014$) and distance travelled (PRE: r = 0.528, $p = 0.016$ and POST: r = 0.568, $p = 0.008$) (Table 4).

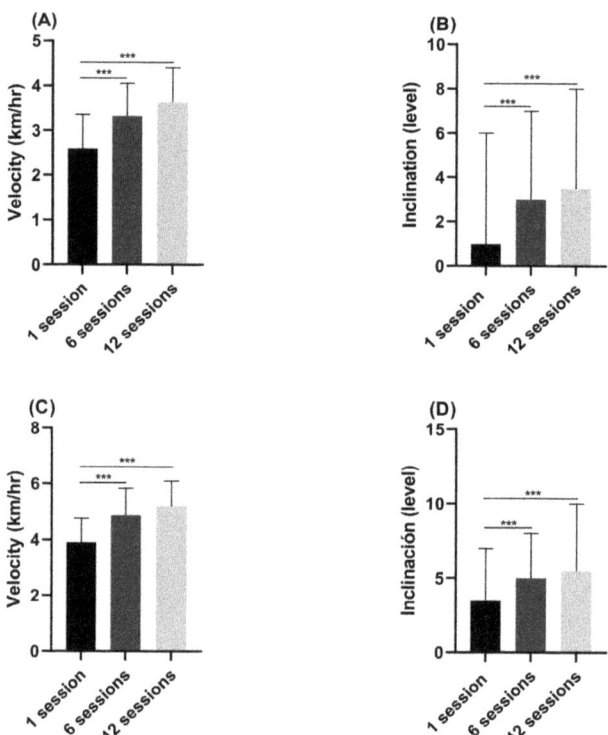

Figure 1. Workloads in pulmonary rehabilitation program sessions. (**A**) Low speed load; (**B**) low tilt load; (**C**) high speed charge; (**D**) high Tilt Load; ***: $p < 0.001$.

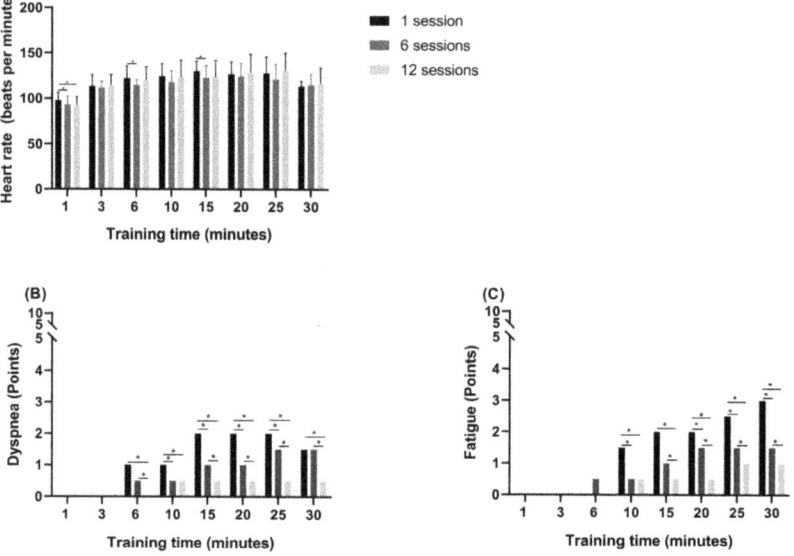

Figure 2. Cardiac response and perceptions in the respiratory rehabilitation program sessions. (**A**) Heart rate; (**B**) dyspnoea; (**C**) fatigue; *: $p < 0.05$.

Table 5. Relationship of the products of heart rate and speed and walked distance in the 6 MWT before and after a pulmonary rehabilitation program.

		PRE	POST
		Correlation p Value	Correlation p Value
HR6 min (bpm)	Velocity (km/h)	0.535 P 0.015	0.555 P 0.011
	Walked distance (m)	0.528 s 0.016	0.613 P 0.011
HRR (bpm)	Velocity (km/h)	0.256 P 0.275	0.421 P 0.064
	Walked distance (m)	0.302 P 0.194	0.461 P 0.040
HR6 min*PS	Velocity (km/h)	0.457 P 0.042	0.538 P 0.014
	Walked distance (m)	0.528 s 0.016	0.568 P 0.008

PRE: before starting the pulmonary rehabilitation program; POST: after the pulmonary rehabilitation program; HR6 min: heart rate at minute 6; HRR: heart rate recovery; bpm: beats per minute; SBP: systolic blood pressure; P: Pearson r coefficient; s: Spearman r coefficient.

7. Discussion

The aim of this research was to analyse the usefulness of HR during the evaluation and development of a pulmonary rehabilitation program in severe COVID-19 patients who survived an MV stay. The main findings were the significant decrease in HRH and the significant increase in HRR after 8 weeks of an individualised and supervised pulmonary rehabilitation program in patients who were severe COVID-19 survivors of MV. There was also a direct and significant relationship between HR6 min, walking speed and walked distance in the 6 MWT, before and after the rehabilitation process. In addition, a significant decrease in the HR of velocity and slope was observed between sessions 1, 6 and 12, accompanied by a significant decrease in the perception of dyspnoea and fatigue. In this line, the importance of this study is that it makes it clear that the beneficial results obtained here reinforce the concept of personalised training.

Gruet et al., set out to determine whether maximal HR during the 6 MWT could be used to predict the gas exchange threshold HR during a maximal cardiopulmonary exercise test in patients with cystic fibrosis. Their results showed that there were no significant differences between HR6 max at 6 MWT and gas exchange threshold HR at maximal cardiopulmonary effort. They also observed a direct and high relationship between the maximum HR in the 6 MWT and the gas exchange threshold HR in both patients with cystic fibrosis ($r = 0.91$; $p = 0.01$) and the control group ($r = 0.81$; $p = 0.01$) [9]. In addition to this, Pepera et al., showed that patients with chronic heart failure have a shorter step length and walk more slowly than controls during the 6 MWT. Altered gait mechanics can contribute to limited exercise capacity in patients with chronic heart failure [29]. This coincides with the results of the present investigation, which indicate that there was a direct and significant relationship between HR6 min and the speed and walked distance in the 6 MWT. Although the HR6 min did not present significant differences after the pulmonary rehabilitation program ($p = 0.381$), the RHR decreased significantly after the pulmonary rehabilitation, a fact that is considered one of the benefits of physical exercise on the cardiac system [13]. This could have "delivered a greater number of heartbeats" at the time of performing the 6 MWT, a fact that could have resulted in a significant increase in speed and distance obtained in the 6 MWT.

On the other hand, the recovery period also showed a significant relationship with the walked distance in the 6 MWT after the pulmonary rehabilitation program. In this regard, Pepera and Panagiota investigated the effects of habitual smoking on heart rate response and HRR after the step test in athletes. Their results indicate that athletes–smokers had a higher RHR ($p < 0.05$) and lower HRR ($p < 0.04$) in relation to athletes–non-smokers. From these results, they concluded that these changes contribute to the adaptation of cardiovascular function to training requirements [30]. On the other hand, Morita et al., compared the physical activity patterns and functional status of COPD participants with or without late recovery of HR after 6 MWT. Their results indicated that patients with a recovery of less than 12 beats/min in the first minute after the end of the 6 MWT have a significant decrease in the walked distance in the 6 MWT versus patients who have a recovery of over 12 beats/min [20]. The present investigation reported a direct and significant relationship between the walked distance and the recovery in the first minute of recovery after the 6 MWT; that is, the greater the beats/min ($\geq$12) of recovery, the greater the distance covered in the 6 MWT. Although it is not possible to identify the cause of the delay in the recovery of HR, Morita et al., linked it to a sedentary lifestyle and decreased ability to exercise [20]. Although the HRR in this investigation only showed a significant relationship with the distance walked after the pulmonary rehabilitation period, this was accompanied by a significant increase in the HRR after the pulmonary rehabilitation program. This could be due to two facts: (i) the best time per turn in the 6 MWT was used to calculate the walking speed, which would not be representative of the behaviour during the entire 6 MWT, and (ii) the training period included forced walking on an incline treadmill and strength exercises, a fact that improved the performance in metres of the 6 MWT; this overload would have allowed cardiac adaptation, resulting in a rapid return to calm. In this context, the HR6 min would be a good indicator of performance in the 6 MWT, which, when complemented with the HRR, would give a complete view of the behaviour of a subject in the face of maximum exercise.

Although there were no significant differences in HR6 min$^\times$SBP after the pulmonary rehabilitation program, direct and significant relationships were observed between HR6 min$^\times$SBP velocity and HR6 min walked distance before and after the pulmonary rehabilitation program. This partially coincides with that reported by Vengatasubramani and Vikram, who investigated the effects of physical training on blood pressure, HR and HR*SBP in COPD participants. The authors studied 30 participants aged between 40 and 55 years; 15 participants were assigned to the experimental group and 15 underwent a pulmonary rehabilitation program consisting of strength exercises. There was a significant difference between the pre- and post-pulmonary rehabilitation values of HR$^\times$SBP (10,270.67 $\pm$ 1379.59 mmHg $\times$ beats/min and 8956.80 $\pm$ 1162.24 mmHg $\times$ beats/min; $p = 0.028$, respectively). This showed that the designed training plan improved cardiovascular fitness in COPD patients [31]. The differences in the results related to HR6 min$^\times$SBP could be due to the series of secondary disorders of COVID-19 in the cardiovascular system [8]. Due to this background, one of the inclusion criteria for the pulmonary rehabilitation program was an electrocardiogram to rule out heart problems.

Although the HR in training increased during the 30 min of forced walking between sessions 1 and 6, it showed a significant decrease in the three evaluations (session 1, session 6 and session 12), despite there being a significant increase in speed and slope. Senanayake et al., investigated the effects of a 6-week pulmonary rehabilitation program on HR response and metabolic demand in patients with pulmonary fibrosis. After the pulmonary rehabilitation program, there was no significant variability in HR pre-exercise ($p = 0.14$) and during exercise ($p = 0.12$). However, it was observed that the HR significantly increased during the recovery state after the intervention ($p = 0.036$). Furthermore, following the pulmonary rehabilitation program, HR variability increased by 68–75% at rest, exercise and during the recovery period [32]. The results of the present investigation also show an increase in HR in the training sessions, accompanied by a significant increase in speed and incline during the pulmonary rehabilitation program. Despite this, the RHR decreased significantly at the end of the pulmonary rehabilitation program, results that would indicate an adaptation to exercise [8,13]. This difference in the final results, between both investigations, could be due to the different basic pathophysiological conditions, where pulmonary fibrosis results in a deterioration that can be progressive and irreversible. In relation to this, Sima et al., showed that high RHR seems to be an indicator of previous myocardial infarction in patients with chronic lung disease; therefore, careful adjustment of training intensity is recommended under these circumstances [33]. Thus, the effect of training would imply the possibility of achieving an adaptation in patients diagnosed with COVID-19. Therefore, there is a need to describe the behaviour of the cardiac system throughout the rehabilitation process of these patients.

Finally, the results show that dyspnoea exhibits the same behaviour as HR during the training sessions (Figure 2A, B). On the other hand, unlike HR, fatigue and dyspnoea increased steadily throughout the training sessions (Figure 2C). The information available indicates that the perception of dyspnoea and fatigue of the lower limbs increases significantly with a higher workload [34]. In addition, perceptions may increase disproportionately during exercise if gas exchange, cardiac output and/or lower limb musculature fail [35]. Thus, a significant decrease in dyspnoea and fatigue accompanied by a decrease in HR could indicate a better adaptation of ventilatory, cardiac and peripheral musculoskeletal function as patients progress through the sessions. Considering the existence of previous reports that indicate the perception of fatigue in 53% and dyspnoea in 43% of post-COVID-19 patients, training within a period of 60 days is important [36].

Future research that could complement the results obtained here would entail observing the impact on quality of life and have more complex measures such as HR variability or VO_{2max}. This research has limitations that need to be discussed. During the critical period of the COVID-19 pandemic, one of the decisions made by the Chilean health authorities was the use of beds in critical units for COVID-19 patients only, so it was not possible to include a control group. This could have generated a potential selection bias. Moreover, the sample of patients studied is low, but it has the strength of being patients who complied with the exercise protocols for 8 weeks and suffered from COVID-19, in addition to being subjected to MV during their illness. The dynamics of health personnel and the redistribution of resources to the closed health system delayed the start of pulmonary rehabilitation, which affected the time of admission to the program. This could have affected the evaluations of lung function and exercise capacity.

8. Conclusions

Eight weeks of an individualised and supervised pulmonary rehabilitation program were effective in improving RHR and HRR in COVID-19 patients who survived MV. HR is an easily accessible indicator that could help to monitor the evaluation and development of a pulmonary rehabilitation program in COVID-19 patients surviving MV.

Author Contributions: Methodology, R.M.-C., C.C.-I., M.F.d.V. and M.d.S.; software, R.M.-C., C.C.-I. and P.A.L.; validation, R.M.-C.; formal analysis, P.A.L. and R.M.-C.; investigation, R.M.-C., P.A.L., M.F.d.V. and J.V.; resources, P.A.L., R.M.-C., M.d.S. and J.V.; data curation, R.M.-C., C.C.-I. and P.A.L.; writing—original draft preparation, G.N.M.-N., R.M.-C., M.d.S., M.F.d.V. and J.V.; writing—review and editing, G.N.M.-N., M.E.-C. and R.M.-C.; visualisation, R.M.-C., M.d.S., M.E.-C. and J.V.; supervision, R.M.-C., G.N.M.-N., M.d.S. and J.V. All authors have read and agreed to the published version of the manuscript.

Funding: This research received no external funding.

Institutional Review Board Statement: This research was approved by the Scientific Ethics Committee of the Central Metropolitan Health Service (Resolution No. 048975, Approval date: 22 June 2021).

Informed Consent Statement: All patients read and signed an informed consent.

Acknowledgments: The authors thank the patients for their willingness to participate in this study.

Conflicts of Interest: The authors declare no conflict of interest.

References

1. MINSAL. Ministerio de Salud de Chile. 120° Informe Epidemiológico Enfermedad por COVID-19 Departamento de Epidemiología. Available online: https://www.minsal.cl/wp-content/uploads/2021/05/Informe-Epidemiolo%CC%81gico-120.pdf (accessed on 19 May 2021).
2. Del Valle, M.F.; Valenzuela, J.; Godoy, L.; Del Sol, M.; Lizana, P.A.; Escobar-Cabello, M.; Munoz-Cofre, R. Letter from Chile. *Respirology* **2021**, *27*, 173–174. [CrossRef] [PubMed]
3. WHO. World Health Organization. Brote De Enfermedad Por Coronavirus (COVID-19). Available online: https://www.who.int/es/emergencies/diseases/novel-coronavirus-2019 (accessed on 19 May 2021).
4. Horton, R. Offline: COVID-19 is not a pandemic. *Lancet* **2020**, *396*, 874. [CrossRef]
5. Wang, T.J.; Chau, B.; Lui, M.; Lam, G.T.; Lin, N.; Humbert, S. Physical Medicine and Rehabilitation and Pulmonary Rehabilitation for COVID-19. *Am. J. Phys. Med. Rehabil.* **2020**, *99*, 769–774. [CrossRef] [PubMed]
6. Alvarez, R.; Del Valle, M.F.; Cordero, P.; Del Sol, M.; Lizana, P.A.; Gutierrez, J.; Valenzuela, P.; Munoz-Cofre, R. Shoulder Pain in COVID-19 Survivors Following Mechanical Ventilation. *Int. J. Environ. Res. Public Health* **2021**, *18*, 10434. [CrossRef] [PubMed]
7. Spruit, M.A.; Holland, A.E.; Singh, S.J.; Tonia, T.; Wilson, K.C.; Troosters, T. COVID-19: Interim Guidance on Rehabilitation in the Hospital and Post-Hospital Phase from a European Respiratory Society and American Thoracic Society-coordinated International Task Force. *Eur. Respir. J.* **2020**, *56*, 2002197. [CrossRef]
8. Chung, M.K.; Zidar, D.A.; Bristow, M.R.; Cameron, S.J.; Chan, T.; Harding, C.V., 3rd; Kwon, D.H.; Singh, T.; Tilton, J.C.; Tsai, E.J.; et al. COVID-19 and Cardiovascular Disease: From Bench to Bedside. *Circ. Res.* **2021**, *128*, 1214–1236. [CrossRef]
9. Gruet, M.; Brisswalter, J.; Mely, L.; Vallier, J.M. Use of the peak heart rate reached during six-minute walk test to predict individualized training intensity in patients with cystic fibrosis: Validity and reliability. *Arch. Phys. Med. Rehabil.* **2010**, *91*, 602–607. [CrossRef]
10. Pepera, G.; Tribali, M.S.; Batalik, L.; Petrov, I.; Papathanasiou, J. Epidemiology, risk factors and prognosis of cardiovascular disease in the Coronavirus Disease 2019 (COVID-19) pandemic era: A systematic review. *Rev. Cardiovasc. Med.* **2022**, *23*, 28. [CrossRef]
11. Gloeckl, R.; Leitl, D.; Jarosch, I.; Schneeberger, T.; Nell, C.; Stenzel, N.; Vogelmeier, C.F.; Kenn, K.; Koczulla, A.R. Benefits of pulmonary rehabilitation in COVID-19: A prospective observational cohort study. *ERJ Open Res.* **2021**, *7*, 00108. [CrossRef]
12. Papathanasiou, G.; Stamou, M.; Stasi, S.; Mamali, A.; Papageorgiou, E. Impact of Physical Activity on Heart Rate, Blood Pressure and Rate-Pressure Product in Healthy Elderly. *Health Sci. J.* **2020**, *14*, 712. [CrossRef]
13. Reimers, A.K.; Knapp, G.; Reimers, C.D. Effects of Exercise on the Resting Heart Rate: A Systematic Review and Meta-Analysis of Interventional Studies. *J. Clin. Med.* **2018**, *7*, 503. [CrossRef] [PubMed]
14. Lindemberg, S.; Chermont, S.; Quintão, M.; Derossi, M.; Guilhon, S.; Bernardez, S.; Marchese, L.; Martins, W.; Nóbrega, A.C.L.; Mesquita, E.T.; et al. Heart Rate Recovery in the First Minute at the Six-Minute Walk Test in Patients with Heart Failure. *Arq. Bras. Cardiol.* **2014**, *102*, 279–287. [CrossRef] [PubMed]
15. Graham, B.L.; Steenbruggen, I.; Miller, M.R.; Barjaktarevic, I.Z.; Cooper, B.G.; Hall, G.L.; Hallstrand, T.S.; Kaminsky, D.A.; McCarthy, K.; McCormack, M.C.; et al. Standardization of Spirometry 2019 Update. An Official American Thoracic Society and European Respiratory Society Technical Statement. *Am. J. Respir. Crit. Care Med.* **2019**, *200*, e70–e88. [CrossRef] [PubMed]
16. SER. Sociedad Chilena de Enfermedades Respiratorias. Recomendación Sobre Pruebas de Función Pulmonar Durante la Pandemia Por Coronavirus COVID-19. Available online: https://serchile.cl/site/docs/recomendacion_PFT.pdf (accessed on 1 June 2021).
17. Miller, M.R.; Hankinson, J.; Brusasco, V.; Burgos, F.; Casaburi, R.; Coates, A.; Crapo, R.; Enright, P.; van der Grinten, C.P.; Gustafsson, P.; et al. Standardisation of spirometry. *Eur. Respir. J.* **2005**, *26*, 319–338. [CrossRef] [PubMed]
18. Muñoz-Cofré, R.; Medina-González, P.; Escobar-Cabello, M. Análisis del comportamiento temporal de variables fisiológicas y de esfuerzo en sujetos instruidos en la Prueba de Caminata en 6 minutos: Complemento a la norma ATS. *Fisioterapia* **2016**, *38*, 20–27. [CrossRef]
19. Borg, G.A. Psychophysical bases of perceived exertion. *Med. Sci. Sports Exerc.* **1982**, *14*, 377–381. [CrossRef]
20. Morita, A.A.; Silva, L.K.O.; Bisca, G.W.; Oliveira, J.M.; Hernandes, N.A.; Pitta, F.; Furlanetto, K.C. Heart Rate Recovery, Physical Activity Level, and Functional Status in Subjects With COPD. *Respir. Care* **2018**, *63*, 1002–1008. [CrossRef]
21. Pinochet, R.; Díaz, O.; Leiva, A.; Borzone, G.; Lisboa, C. Adaptación de la prueba de marcha de 6 minutos en corredor a cinta rodante en pacientes con enfermedad pulmonar obstructiva crónica. *Rev. Kinesiol.* **2003**, *72*, 69–72.
22. Northridge, D.B.; Grant, S.; Ford, I.; Christie, J.; McLenachan, J.; Connelly, D.; McMurray, J.; Ray, S.; Henderson, E.; Dargie, H.J. Novel exercise protocol suitable for use on a treadmill or a bicycle ergometer. *Br. Heart J.* **1990**, *64*, 313–316. [CrossRef]
23. Killian, K.J.; Leblanc, P.; Martin, D.H.; Summers, E.; Jones, N.L.; Campbell, E.J. Exercise capacity and ventilatory, circulatory, and symptom limitation in patients with chronic airflow limitation. *Am. Rev. Respir. Dis.* **1992**, *146*, 935–940. [CrossRef]
24. Romer, L. Cardiopulmonary exercise testing in patients with ventilatory disorders. In *Sport and Exercise Physiology Testing Guidelines: Volume II-Exercise and Clinical Testing*; Edward, M., Winter, A.M.J., Davison, R.R.C., Bromley, P.D., Mercer, T., Eds.; Routledge: Londres, UK; New York, NY, USA, 2007; Volume 2, pp. 179–188.
25. López, R.C.-V.P.; Devaud, Y.; Muñoz-Cofré, R.; Gómez-Bruton, A.; Lizana, P.A. Can elastic band resistance training programs mitigate holiday weight gain and improve hand-grip strength in older women? *Int. J. Morphol.* **2020**, *38*, 1173–1178. [CrossRef]
26. Kim, S.Y.; Busch, A.J.; Overend, T.J.; Schachter, C.L.; van der Spuy, I.; Boden, C.; Goes, S.M.; Foulds, H.J.; Bidonde, J. Flexibility exercise training for adults with fibromyalgia. *Cochrane Database Syst. Rev.* **2019**, *9*, CD013419. [CrossRef] [PubMed]

27. Hawkins, S.W.; Hawkins, J.R. Clinical Applications of Cryotherapy Among Sports Physical Therapists. *Int. J. Sports Phys. Ther.* **2016**, *11*, 141–148. [PubMed]
28. Ferraro, F.V.; Gavin, J.P.; Wainwright, T.; McConnell, A. The effects of 8 weeks of inspiratory muscle training on the balance of healthy older adults: A randomized, double-blind, placebo-controlled study. *Physiol. Rep.* **2019**, *7*, e14076. [CrossRef] [PubMed]
29. Pepera, G.; Sandercock, G.R.; Sloan, R.; Cleland, J.; Ingle, L.; Clark, A. Influence of step length on 6-minute walk test performance in patients with chronic heart failure. *Physiotherapy* **2012**, *98*, 325–329. [CrossRef]
30. Pepera, G.; Panagiota, Z. Comparison of heart rate response and heart rate recovery after step test among smoker and non-smoker athletes. *Afri. Health Sci.* **2021**, *21*, 105–111. [CrossRef]
31. Vengatasubramani, M.; Vikram, M. Physical Training Improved Cardiovascular Fitness Level among Chronic Obstructive Pulmonary Disease Patients. *Med. Health* **2014**, *9*, 109–113.
32. Senanayake, S.; Harrison, N.; Lewis, M. Influence of physical rehabilitation on heart rate dynamics in patients with idiopathic pulmonary fibrosis. *J. Exerc. Rehabil.* **2019**, *15*, 160–169. [CrossRef]
33. Sima, C.; Lau, B.C.; Taylor, C.M.; van Eeden, S.F.; Reid, W.D.; Sheel, A.W.; Kirkham, A.R.; Camp, P. Myocardial Infarction Injury in Patients with Chronic Lung Disease Entering Pulmonary Rehabilitation: Frequency and Association with Heart Rate Parameters. *PM R* **2018**, *10*, 917–925. [CrossRef]
34. Satia, I.; Farooqi, M.A.M.; Cusack, R.; Matsuoka, M.; Yanqing, X.; Kurmi, O.; O'Byrne, P.M.; Killian, K.J. The contribution of FEV_1 and airflow limitation on the intensity of dyspnea and leg effort during exercise. Insights from a real-world cohort. *Physiol. Rep.* **2020**, *8*, e14415. [CrossRef]
35. Garcia-Rio, F.; Rojo, B.; Casitas, R.; Lores, V.; Madero, R.; Romero, D.; Galera, R.; Villasante, C. Prognostic value of the objective measurement of daily physical activity in patients with COPD. *Chest* **2012**, *142*, 338–346. [CrossRef] [PubMed]
36. Sigfrid, L.; Cevik, M.; Jesudason, E.; Lim, W.S.; Rello, J.; Amuasi, J.; Bozza, F.; Palmieri, C.; Munblit, D.; Holter, J.C.; et al. What is the recovery rate and risk of long-term consequences following a diagnosis of COVID-19? A harmonised, global longitudinal observational study protocol. *BMJ Open* **2021**, *11*, e043887. [CrossRef] [PubMed]

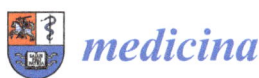

Communication

COVID-19 Pneumonia in Fully Vaccinated Adults during the Dominance of the Omicron Sublineages BA.1.1 and BA.2 in Mexico

Efrén Murillo-Zamora [1,2], Xóchitl Trujillo [3], Miguel Huerta [3], Mónica Riós-Silva [4], José Guzmán-Esquivel [2,5], Jaime Alberto Bricio-Barrios [2], Oliver Mendoza-Cano [6,*] and Agustin Lugo-Radillo [7,*]

1. Departamento de Epidemiología, Unidad de Medicina Familiar No. 19, Instituto Mexicano del Seguro Social, Av. Javier Mina 301, Col. Centro, Colima 28000, Mexico
2. Facultad de Medicina, Universidad de Colima, Av. Universidad 333, Col. Las Víboras, Colima 28040, Mexico
3. Centro Universitario de Investigaciones Biomédicas, Universidad de Colima, Av. 25 de julio 965, Col. Villas San Sebastián, Colima 28045, Mexico
4. Centro Universitario de Investigaciones Biomédicas, Universidad de Colima-CONACyT, Av. 25 de julio 965, Col. Villas de San Sebastián, Colima 28045, Mexico
5. Unidad de Investigación en Epidemiología Clínica, Hospital General de Zona No. 1, Instituto Mexicano del Seguro Social, Av. Lapislázuli 250, Col. El Haya, Villa de Álvarez, Colima 28984, Mexico
6. Facultad de Ingeniería Civil, Universidad de Colima, km. 9 Carretera Colima-Coquimatlán, Coquimatlán, Colima 28400, Mexico
7. CONACYT—Faculty of Medicine and Surgery, Universidad Autónoma Benito Juárez de Oaxaca, Oaxaca 68020, Mexico
* Correspondence: oliver@ucol.mx (O.M.-C.); alugora@conacyt.mx (A.L.-R.); Tel.: +52-312-316-1167 (O.M.-C.)

Abstract: *Background and Objectives:* A nationwide retrospective cohort study was conducted to evaluate the factors associated with the risk of laboratory-confirmed coronavirus disease 2019 (COVID-19)-related pneumonia in fully vaccinated adults during the dominance of the Omicron sublineages in Mexico. *Materials and Methods:* Fully COVID-19-vaccinated adults with laboratory-positive illness and symptom onset from April to mid-June 2022 were eligible. We computed the eta-squared (η^2) to evaluate the effect size of the study sample. The characteristics predicting pneumonia were evaluated through risk ratios (RRs), and the 95% confidence intervals (CIs) were computed through generalized linear models. *Results:* The data from 35,561 participants were evaluated, and the overall risk of pneumonia was 0.5%. In multiple analyses, patients aged $\geq$ 60 years old were at increased risk of developing pneumonia (vs. 20–39 years old: RR = 1.031, 95% CI = 1.027–1.034). Chronic pulmonary obstructive disease, type 2 diabetes mellitus, arterial hypertension, chronic kidney disease (any stage), and immunosuppression (any cause) were also associated with a higher pneumonia risk. The η^2 of all the variables included in the multiple models was <0.06. *Conclusions:* Our study suggests that, even when fully COVID-19-vaccinated, older adults and those with chronic conditions were at increased risk of pneumonia during the dominance of the Omicron sublineages BA.1.1 and BA.2.

Keywords: COVID-19 vaccines; adult; pneumonia; risk

Citation: Murillo-Zamora, E.; Trujillo, X.; Huerta, M.; Riós-Silva, M.; Guzmán-Esquivel, J.; Bricio-Barrios, J.A.; Mendoza-Cano, O.; Lugo-Radillo, A. COVID-19 Pneumonia in Fully Vaccinated Adults during the Dominance of the Omicron Sublineages BA.1.1 and BA.2 in Mexico. *Medicina* 2022, 58, 1127. https://doi.org/10.3390/medicina58081127

Academic Editor: Masaki Okamoto

Received: 16 July 2022
Accepted: 15 August 2022
Published: 19 August 2022

Publisher's Note: MDPI stays neutral with regard to jurisdictional claims in published maps and institutional affiliations.

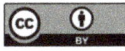

Copyright: © 2022 by the authors. Licensee MDPI, Basel, Switzerland. This article is an open access article distributed under the terms and conditions of the Creative Commons Attribution (CC BY) license (https://creativecommons.org/licenses/by/4.0/).

1. Introduction

In Mexico, the vaccination efforts against coronavirus disease 2019 (COVID-19) in the general population started early in 2021. By the first week of June 2022, about 61% of inhabitants had been fully vaccinated [1].

According to genomic sequencing data, the sublineages BA.2 (B.1.1.529.2) and BA.1.1 (also known as BA.1 + R346K of the Omicron variant (B.1.1.529)) were dominating in Mexican territory from April to mid-June 2022 [2]. These strains were identified in 71% and 23% of sequenced cases [2]. Recently published in vitro evidence suggests that the BA.1.1 and BA.2 sublineages are antigenically equidistant from wild-type SARS-CoV-2, and thus, similarly threaten the efficacy of first-generation vaccines [3].

This study aimed to identify the factors associated with the risk of COVID-19-related pneumonia in fully vaccinated adults during the Omicron sublineages BA.1.1 and BA.2 in Mexico.

2. Materials and Methods

We performed a nationwide retrospective cohort study in Mexico during the first half of July 2022. The potentially eligible subjects were fully vaccinated (at least two shots from any COVID-19 vaccine) adults (aged 20 years or older) with laboratory-confirmed (reverse transcription–polymerase chain reaction (RT-PCR) or rapid antigen test via nasal swabbing) COVID-19. Patients with illness onset from 1 April to 15 June 2022 were eligible, and they were identified from the records of a normative system for the epidemiological surveillance of respiratory viral diseases of the Mexican Institute of Social Security (with the Spanish acronym IMSS). Subjects with more than 12 months between the date of the second vaccine shot and the date of illness onset were excluded.

A broader description of the employed laboratory methods was published elsewhere [4,5]. The clinical and epidemiological data of interest were retrieved from the audited surveillance system. The main binary (no/yes) outcome was pneumonia, and it was defined by the presence of clinical (cough, dyspnea, and fever) radiographic (ground-glass opacities from computed tomography scan or chest X-ray) findings in patients with laboratory-positive COVID-19 who required hospital admission [6].

Summary statistics were computed, and generalized linear regression models were used to estimate the risk ratios (RRs) and 95% confidence intervals (CIs). We assessed the eta-squared (η^2) of the multiple models to evaluate the effect size of the study sample. The analytical procedure was performed using the statistical package Stata MP 14.0 (StataCorp; College Station, TX, USA).

3. Results

The data from 35,561 patients were analyzed and the overall risk of pneumonia was 0.5% (n = 162/35,561). Most of the participants were female (58.4%), and their mean age (±standard deviation) was 38.2 ± 12.9 years (total range: 20 to 90 years). The mortality risk among patients with pneumonia was 27.8% (n = 45/162).

The mean interval between the last vaccine shot and the date of symptom onset was 8.3 ± 3.2 months. About 7 out of 10 of the enrolled patients received the Vaxzevria (38.8%; ChAdOx1, AstraZeneca, Cambridge, UK) or BNT162b2 (28.4%; Pfizer-BioNTech, Mainz, Germany) COVID-19 vaccines.

When compared with patients with mild COVID-19 symptoms, those with pneumonia were older (61.4 ± 17.3 vs. 38.1 ± 12.8 years, p < 0.001) and had a higher prevalence of obesity (body mass index equal to or higher than 30, 17.3% vs. 9.0%, p < 0.001), previously diagnosed chronic pulmonary obstructive disease (7.4% vs. 0.4%, p < 0.001), type 2 diabetes mellitus (42.6% vs. 6.1%, p < 0.001), arterial hypertension (54.3% vs. 10.3%, p < 0.001), chronic kidney disease (any stage; 22.2% vs. 0.5%, p < 0.001) and immunosuppression (any cause excepting type 2 diabetes mellitus; 5.6% vs. 0.4%, p < 0.001). No significant differences were observed between the study groups in terms gender and tobacco use (current).

In the multiple analysis (Table 1) and when compared with younger subjects (20–39 years old), patients aged 60 years or above were at increased risk of pneumonia (RR = 1.031, 95% CI = 1.027–1.034). The highest increase in pneumonia risk was documented in patients with chronic kidney disease (any stage; RR = 1.146, 95% CI = 1.136–1.156). Type 2 diabetes mellitus, arterial hypertension, and immunosuppression were also associated with an increased risk of developing pneumonia. The η^2 of all the variables included in the multiple models (Table 1) was <0.06, so the effect size may be considered small–medium.

Table 1. Predictors of pneumonia in laboratory-confirmed COVID-19 among fully vaccinated adults during the dominance of the Omicron sublineages, Mexico, 2022.

Characteristic	RR (95% CI), p			
	Bivariate Analysis		Multiple Analysis	
Gender				
Female	1.000		1.000	
Male	1.001 (0.999–1.003),	0.090	1.001 (0.999–1.002),	0.152
Age group (years)				
20–39	1.000		1.000	
40–59	1.003 (1.001–1.004),	<0.001	1.001 (0.998–1.002),	0.718
60 or above	1.042 (1.039–1.045),	<0.001	1.031 (1.027–1.034),	<0.001
Months elapsed from the last vaccine shot to illness onset				
<6	1.000		1.000	
6 or above	1.004 (1.002–1.005),	<0.001	1.001 (0.999–1.002),	0.363
Personal history of:				
Obesity (BMI of 30 or above)				
No	1.000		1.000	
Yes	1.005 (1.002–1.007),	<0.001	1.001 (0.998–1.003),	0.458
Chronic pulmonary obstructive disease				
No	1.000		1.000	
Yes	1.082 (1.070–1.094),	<0.001	1.049 (1.038–1.060),	<0.001
Type 2 diabetes mellitus				
No	1.000		1.000	
Yes	1.028 (1.026–1.031),	<0.001	1.014 (1.011–1.017),	<0.001
Arterial hypertension				
No	1.000		1.000	
Yes	1.022 (1.019–1.024),	<0.001	1.005 (1.002–1.007),	<0.001
Chronic kidney disease (any stage)				
No	1.000		1.000	
Yes	1.169 (1.158–1.179),	<0.001	1.146 (1.136–1.156),	<0.001
Immunosuppression				
No	1.000		1.000	
Yes	1.059 (1.047–1.070),	<0.001	1.036 (1.026–1.048),	<0.001

Abbreviations: COVID-19—coronavirus disease 2019; RR—risk ratio; CI—confidence interval. Notes: (1) Generalized linear regression models were used to compute the RR and 95% CI; (2) the estimates from the multiple analysis were adjusted by all the variables presented in the table; (3) immunosuppression refers to any cause of the inhibition of the normal immune response, excepting those related to type 2 diabetes mellitus.

4. Discussion

Our study evaluated the factors predicting COVID-19-related pneumonia in fully vaccinated adults and during the dominance of the Omicron sublineages BA.1.1 and BA.2 in Mexico. We identified populations at risk that may benefit from specific interventions focusing on reducing the transmission of viral respiratory pathogens.

We found that increasing age seems to be an independent risk factor for pneumonia, even in fully immunized adults. However, the risk of severe manifestations among elderly subjects (aged 60 years or above) in our study was 4.2% ($n = 96/2177$), which is considerably lower than the risk observed during the dominance of the wild-type strain and which was as high as 60% [7].

A lower antibody response after vaccination has been documented in older individuals [8]. In addition, the interval between the date of the most recent vaccination and the date of symptom onset was higher among elderly participants. This latter was due to the prioritization of older adults at the start of vaccination efforts in the general population. We consider that these two aspects may be determined, at least partially, by the observed scenario among aged participants.

The association between chronic comorbidities and the risk of pneumonia in COVID-19 has been largely known [9]. In our study sample, the highest risk (RR = 1.146, 95%

CI = 1.136–1.156) was documented in a patient with a personal history of chronic kidney disease (any stage), which shows epidemic characteristics in Mexico [10].

According to the most recent local guidelines, molecular testing for COVID-19 is performed only in cases requiring non-ambulatory management. A positive RT-PCR was available for 3.2% (n = 1130) of participants (all of them had pneumonia); the remaining analyzed cases were confirmed using antigen-based testing.

We lacked genomic sequencing data for all the analyzed individuals, which represents a significant limitation of the study. However, according to the official data from the General Directorate of Epidemiology of Mexico, the dominance of the two analyzed sublineages was clear, and it agrees with a growing trend in the number of confirmed cases throughout the Mexican territory. In addition, we only analyzed fully vaccinated subjects and, therefore, we were unable to assess the risk of COVID-19-related pneumonia in non-vaccinated adults.

5. Conclusions

We characterized the risk of COVID-19-related pneumonia in a large set of fully vaccinated adults during the dominance of the Omicron sublineages BA.1.1 and BA.2. We identified the populations at risk that may benefit from maintaining more strict non-pharmaceutical interventions against COVID-19, even if they are fully vaccinated.

Author Contributions: Conceptualization, E.M.-Z. and O.M-C.; data curation, J.G.-E. and J.A.B.-B.; investigation, X.T., M.H., J.G.-E. and M.R.-S.; methodology, A.L.-R.; software, J.A.B.-B. and M.R.-S.; supervision, M.H.; validation, X.T.; visualization, M.R.-S.; writing—original draft, E.M.-Z. and O.M.-C.; writing—review and editing, O.M.-C., M.R.-S. and A.L.-R. All authors have read and agreed to the published version of the manuscript.

Funding: This research received no external funding.

Institutional Review Board Statement: The Local Health Research Ethics Committee (601) of the IMSS approved this research protocol (R-2020-601-015) wherein fully anonymized data were used.

Informed Consent Statement: Not applicable.

Data Availability Statement: All data can be made available upon request to the corresponding authors.

Acknowledgments: The group of researchers would like to thank the Mexican Institute of Social Security for the data provided and for their valuable support in the development of this research.

Conflicts of Interest: The authors declare no conflict of interest.

References

1. Oxford University. Our World in Data: Coronavirus (COVID-19) Vaccinations (Updated on 9 June 2022). Available online: https://ourworldindata.org/covid-vaccinations (accessed on 10 July 2022).
2. General Directorate of Epidemiology of Mexico. Genomic Surveillance Report of the SARS-CoV-2 Virus in Mexico National and State Distribution of Variants as of 16 May 2022. Available online: https://coronavirus.gob.mx/wp-content/uploads/2022/05/2022.05.16-Variantes-COVID-MX.pdf (accessed on 10 July 2022).
3. Iketani, S.; Liu, L.; Guo, Y.; Liu, L.; Chan, J.F.-W.; Huang, Y.; Wang, M.; Luo, Y.; Yu, J.; Chu, H.; et al. Antibody evasion properties of SARS-CoV-2 Omicron sublineages. *Nature* **2022**, *604*, 553–556. [CrossRef] [PubMed]
4. Murillo-Zamora, E.; Trujillo, X.; Huerta, M.; Ríos-Silva, M.; Mendoza-Cano, O. Performance of Antigen-Based Testing as Frontline Diagnosis of Symptomatic COVID-19. *Medicina* **2021**, *57*, 852. [CrossRef] [PubMed]
5. Murillo-Zamora, E.; Trujillo, X.; Huerta, M.; Ríos-Silva, M.; Mendoza-Cano, O. Male gender and kidney illness are associated with an increased risk of severe laboratory-confirmed coronavirus disease. *BMC Infect. Dis.* **2020**, *20*, 674. [CrossRef] [PubMed]
6. Landini, N.; Orlandi, M.; Fusaro, M.; Ciet, P.; Nardi, C.; Bertolo, S.; Catalanotti, V.; Matucci-Cerinic, M.; Colagrande, S.; Morana, G. The Role of Imaging in COVID-19 Pneumonia Diagnosis and Management: Main Positions of the Experts, Key Imaging Features and Open Answers. *J. Cardiovasc. Echogr.* **2020**, *30* (Suppl. 2), S25–S30. [PubMed]
7. Dhama, K.; Patel, S.K.; Kumar, R.; Rana, J.; Yatoo, M.I.; Kumar, A.; Tiwari, R.; Dhama, J.; Natesan, S.; Singh, R.; et al. Geriatric Population During the COVID-19 Pandemic: Problems, Considerations, Exigencies, and Beyond. *Front. Public Health* **2020**, *8*, 574198. [CrossRef] [PubMed]
8. Anastassopoulou, C.; Antoni, D.; Manoussopoulos, Y.; Stefanou, P.; Argyropoulou, S.; Vrioni, G.; Tsakris, A. Age and sex associations of SARS-CoV-2 antibody responses post BNT162b2 vaccination in healthcare workers: A mixed effects model across two vaccination periods. *PLoS ONE* **2022**, *17*, e0266958. [CrossRef] [PubMed]

9. Gimeno-Miguel, A.; Bliek-Bueno, K.; Poblador-Plou, B.; Carmona-Pírez, J.; Poncel-Falcó, A.; González-Rubio, F.; Ioakeim-Skoufa, I.; Pico-Soler, V.; Aza-Pascual-Salcedo, M.; Prados-Torres, A.; et al. Chronic diseases associated with increased likelihood of hospitalization and mortality in 68,913 COVID-19 confirmed cases in Spain: A population-based cohort study. *PLoS ONE* **2021**, *16*, e0259822. [CrossRef] [PubMed]
10. Agudelo-Botero, M.; Valdez-Ortiz, R.; Giraldo-Rodríguez, L.; González-Robledo, M.C.; Mino-León, D.; Rosales-Herrera, M.F.; Cahuana-Hurtado, L.; Rojas-Russell, M.E.; Dávila-Cervantes, C.A. Overview of the burden of chronic kidney disease in Mexico: Secondary data analysis based on the Global Burden of Disease Study 2017. *BMJ Open* **2020**, *10*, e035285. [CrossRef] [PubMed]

Case Report

Pneumocystis jirovecii Pneumonia Associated with COVID-19 in Patients with Interstitial Pneumonia

Tomoyuki Takahashi [†], Atsushi Saito [†], Koji Kuronuma *, Hirotaka Nishikiori and Hirofumi Chiba

Department of Respiratory Medicine and Allergology, Sapporo Medical University School of Medicine, Sapporo 060-8543, Japan
* Correspondence: kuronumak@sapmed.ac.jp
† These authors contributed equally to this work.

Abstract: Here, we report two cases of patients with interstitial pneumonia (IP) on steroids who developed *Pneumocystis jirovecii* pneumonia (PJP) following coronavirus disease 2019 (COVID-19) infection. Case 1: A 69-year-old man on 10 mg of prednisolone (PSL) daily for IP developed new pneumonia shortly after his COVID-19 infection improved and was diagnosed with PJP based on chest computed tomography (CT) findings and elevated serum β-D-glucan levels. Trimethoprim–sulfamethoxazole (TMP–SMZ) was administered, and the pneumonia resolved. Case 2: A 70-year-old woman taking 4 mg/day of PSL for IP and rheumatoid arthritis developed COVID-19 pneumonia, which resolved mildly, but her pneumonia flared up and was diagnosed as PJP based on CT findings, elevated β-D-glucan levels, and positive polymerase chain reaction for *P. jirovecii* DNA in the sputum. The autopsy revealed diffuse alveolar damage, increased collagen fiver and fibrotic foci, mucinous component accumulation, and the presence of a *P. jirovecii* cyst. In conclusion, steroids and immunosuppressive medications are well-known risk factors for PJP. Patients with IP who have been taking these drugs for a long time are frequently treated with additional steroids for COVID-19; thus, PJP complications should be avoided in such cases.

Keywords: SARS-CoV-2; COVID-19; *Pneumocystis jirovecii* pneumonia; interstitial pneumonia; steroids; immunosuppressive drugs

1. Introduction

Except for idiopathic pulmonary fibrosis in the chronic phase, the use of steroids and immunosuppressive agents is often considered for treating other interstitial pneumonias [1]. Steroids are also often used in COVID-19 pneumonia to control the excessive inflammation associated with viral infections [2]. One of the most important factors to consider when using these drugs is the rise in infections associated with immunodeficiency [3]. *Pneumocystis jirovecii* pneumonia (PJP) is one such disease wherein immunosuppression is a risk factor and has a significant impact on prognosis. Therefore, patients with interstitial pneumonia (IP) taking steroids or immunosuppressive medications should be approached with caution. We present two cases of PJP at our institution, both of which occurred after COVID-19 infection in patients with IP on steroids.

2. Case Report

2.1. Case 1

A 69-year-old man diagnosed with IP in 2018 and receiving oral prednisolone (PSL) at a maintenance dose of 10 mg daily developed a fever in April 2020, and the polymerase chain reaction (PCR) test was positive for SARS-CoV2. He had not received the COVID-19 vaccine. Treatment began with oral favipiravir, which was widely used for COVID-19 treatment in Japan at the time. However, due to the patient's lack of improvement and poor oxygenation, he was admitted to our hospital on the seventh day after his illness began. Upon examination, his body temperature was 36.2 °C, his heart rate was 51 beats/min, and his oxygen saturation was 94% (room air). The blood examination showed the following results: white blood cells (WBC) $30.1 \times 10^3/\mu L$, hemoglobin (Hb) 14.8 g/dL, platelets $45.8 \times 10^4/\mu L$, Na 136 mEq/L, K 4.2 mEq/L, Cl 97 mEq/L, C-reactive protein (CRP) 0.75 mg/dL, blood urea nitrogen (BUN) 23 mg/dL, creatinine (Cre) 0.88 mg/dL, aspartate aminotransferase (AST) 72 IU/L, alanine aminotransferase (ALT) 92 IU/L, and lactate dehydrogenase (LDH) 370 U/L. These findings are typical in the early stages of COVID-19 infection. Figure 1A depicts the patient's clinical course. Ground-glass opacities and consolidation were seen on chest computed tomography (CT) (Figure 2). COVID-19 pneumonia was almost completely resolved after the fever subsided. The patient developed fever again on the 19th day after the onset of the disease (Day 19), and a chest CT scan revealed a new ground-glass opacity (GGO), thereby raising the possibility of pneumonia caused by a common bacterium. Levofloxacin treatment was ineffective, and an increase in serum β-D-glucan levels to 9.7 pg/mL increased the possibility of PJP. The fact that trimethoprim–sulfamethoxazole (TMP–SMZ) improved pneumonia led to a clinical diagnosis of PJP.

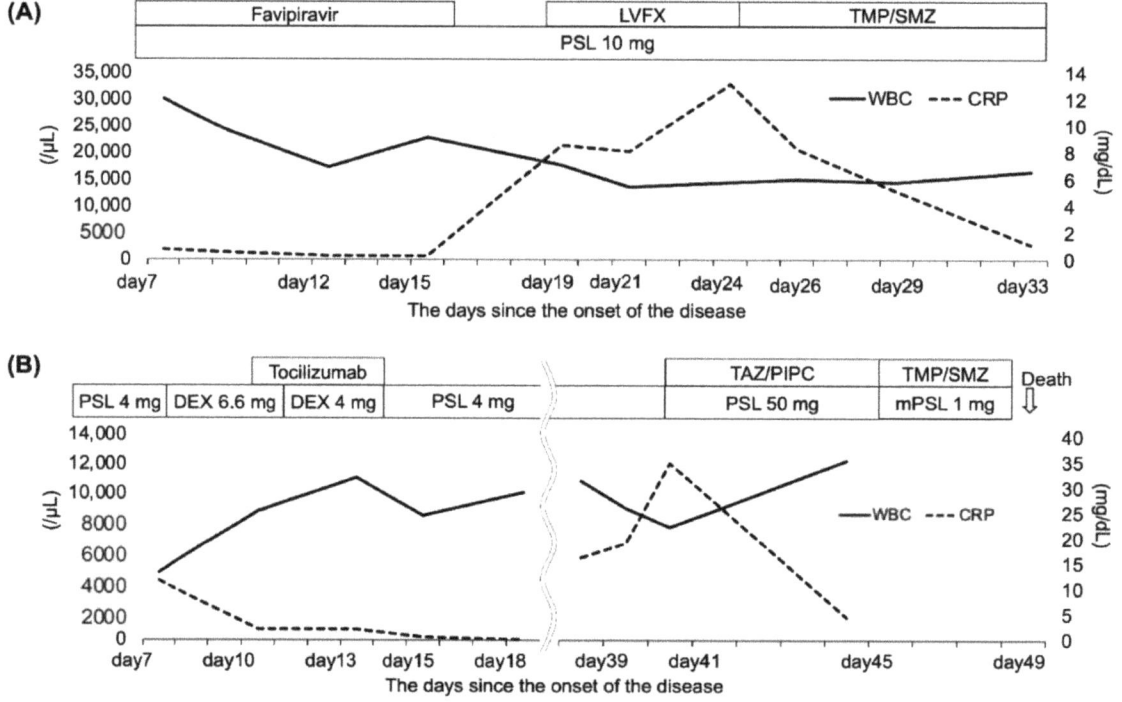

Figure 1. The clinical course of the patients. (**A**) case 1. (**B**) case 2. WBC: white blood cell, CPR: C-reactive protein, PSL: prednisolone, DEX: dexamethasone, LVFX: Levofloxacin, TMP/SMX: trimethoprim/sulfamethoxazole, TAZ/PIPC: tazobactam/piperacillin.

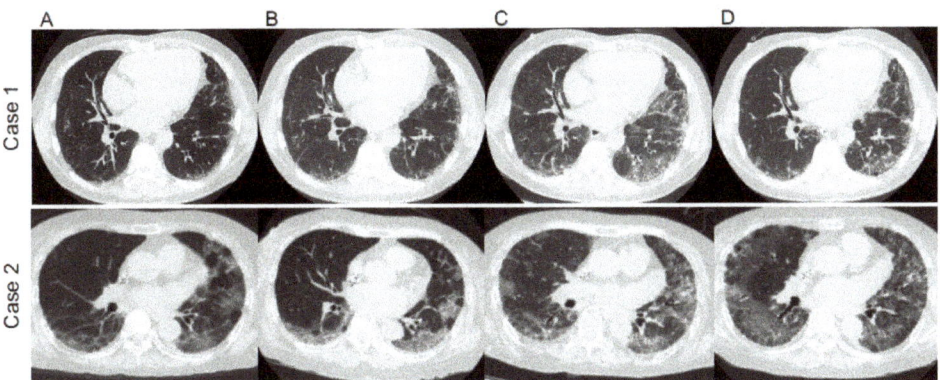

Figure 2. Chest computed tomography (CT) images of Case 1 and Case 2 (**A**) at COVID-19 diagnosis, (**B**) after treatment of COVID-19, (**C**) at *Pneumocystis jirovecii* pneumonia (PJP) diagnosis, and (**D**) after PJP treatment with trimethoprim–sulfamethoxazole.

2.2. Case 2

A 70-year-old woman taking 4 mg of PSL orally daily for IP and rheumatoid arthritis was admitted to our hospital in April 2021 for COVID-19 treatment for 18 days (Days 7–25), where dexamethasone and tocilizumab were used. She had not received the COVID-19 vaccine. She began coughing one week after discharge (day 33), and five days later, she developed respiratory failure, with a chest CT revealing worsening pneumonia. Therefore, she was readmitted to the hospital (Day 38). During the second examination, her body temperature was 36.3 °C, her heart rate was 91 beats/min, and her oxygen saturation was 94% (2 L/min). The blood examination showed the following results: WBC $11.0 \times 10^3/\mu L$, Hb 12.0 g/dL, platelets $14 \times 10^4/\mu L$, Na 123 mEq/L, K 4.5 mEq/L, Cl 90 mEq/L, CRP 16.24 mg/dL, BUN 16 mg/dL, Cre 0.57 mg/dL, AST 23 IU/L, ALT 12 IU/L, and LDH 438 U/L. At this time, the quantitative SARS-CoV-2 antigen test was negative. Figure 1B depicts the patient's clinical course. Her respiratory failure worsened after admission, her serum CRP was elevated, and a chest CT revealed an enlarged GGO (Figure 2). Ultimately, the diagnosis of PJP was made on the basis of high serum β-D-glucan levels and positive PCR for *P. jirovecii* DNA in the sputum. Thus, she was given TMP–SMZ treatment, but her respiratory failure worsened and she died on Day 49. She was subjected to a pathological autopsy. The lungs were clogged, and the histological assessment revealed multiple diffuse vitreous membranes, a sign of diffuse alveolar damage (DAD). Her collagen fiber increased in the interstitium, and numerous fibroblast foci were found in the alveolar wall and space. Furthermore, there was mucinous and exudate accumulation in the interstitium and alveolar space (Figure 3). Additionally, *P. jirovecii* cyst was identified. Although COVID-19 pneumonia and acute exacerbation of IP could cause DAD, PJP was determined to be the cause based on clinical and laboratory findings.

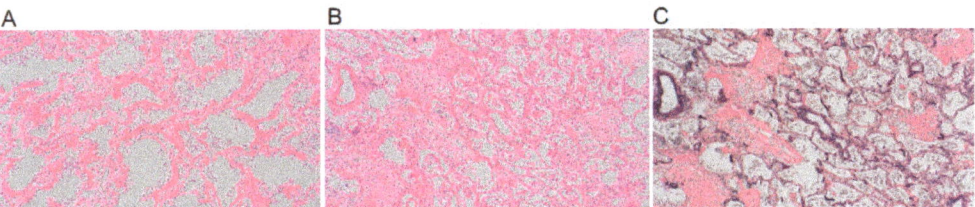

Figure 3. The lung sections obtained from autopsy were stained with the hematoxylin–eosin stain (**A**,**B**) and the Elastica van Gieson stain (**C**). Representative images of (**A**) hyaline membranes' line alveolar spaces, (**B**) fibroblastic foci, and (**C**) fibrotic lung tissue are shown (original magnification × 200).

3. Discussion

The differential diagnosis of post-COVID-19 pneumonia should include COVID-19 pneumonia relapse, acute exacerbation of IP [4], secondary infectious pneumonia [5–7], and organizing pneumonia [8]. Here, PJP was diagnosed based on the CT findings, the elevated serum β-D-glucan levels, and a positive PCR test for *P. jiroveci* DNA in the sputum.

According to many reports, complications of bacterial infection and secondary infections are uncommon after COVID-19 pneumonia. Furthermore, there have been a few reports of PJP following COVID-19 infection [9], but there is currently no consensus. Some cytokines are known to affect not only the control of infections but also fibrosis of the lungs. Zhong JH et al. reported that lower circulating interferon-gamma is a risk factor for lung fibrosis in patients with COVID-19 infections [10]. There is also a report of cytokine-mediated involvement of tuberculosis and helminth infection in pulmonary fibrosis secondary to COVID-19 [11]. Although the involvement of cytokines in PJP after COVID-19 pneumonia with IP has not been investigated, there is room for further studies on this matter. Additionally, both cases in this study were non-vaccinated cases. A comparison of the risk of PJP in COVID-19 pneumonia between patients who are vaccinated and non-vaccinated is also the subject of a future study. Corticosteroids are recommended for treating COVID-19 pneumonia when respiratory failure due to the pathogenesis of acute respiratory disease syndrome (ARDS) becomes severe [2], but caution should be exercised because of the risk of developing PJP in some patients, as in these cases. During the two years from February 2020 to January 2022, 11 patients (1.1%) admitted to and treated at our hospital had underlying IP. Because we were unable to follow up with all of the patients, these data are only for reference purposes; however, the two cases shown here were those who developed PJP after their infection with COVID-19 was cured. Given that PJP was observed in two of the eleven patients with IP who had previously received steroid treatment, we believe that special attention should be paid to the development of PJP in patients with COVID-19 receiving steroid treatment for IP. There has been no pathological autopsy report of a case of PJP in a patient with IP after COVID-19 infection, and this is the first such case. Lesions primarily composed of DAD were found in the lungs. Along with the original IP lesions, the combination of ARDS-like effusion in the alveolar space caused by COVID-19 and an infectious lesion caused by PJP was the reason for the unfavorable outcome of this case. Although the number of patients presenting with pneumonia such as this case has decreased since Omicron strains became the mainstay of COVID-19 infection, we believe that these two cases highlight the importance of being cautious about secondary PJP development in the future.

4. Conclusions

In conclusion, using steroids and immunosuppressive medications increases the risk of developing PJP. However, since patients with IP who have been taking these medications for a long time frequently receive additional steroid treatment for COVID-19 pneumonia, we should be especially watchful for PJP complications in these situations.

Author Contributions: A.S. and K.K. developed the study design. T.T. and A.S. analyzed and interpreted the data and wrote the manuscript. H.N. and H.C. assisted with data analysis and interpretation and supervised the analysis. All authors have read and agreed to the published version of the manuscript.

Funding: This research received no external funding.

Institutional Review Board Statement: No specific ethics committee approval was required for this study.

Informed Consent Statement: Written informed consent was obtained from the patient or patient's family to publish this paper.

Data Availability Statement: Data supporting the study findings are available from the corresponding author upon reasonable request.

Acknowledgments: Not applicable.

Conflicts of Interest: The authors declare no conflict of interest.

References

1. Raghu, G.; Remy-Jardin, M.; Richeldi, L.; Thomson, C.C.; Inoue, Y.; Johkoh, T.; Kreuter, M.; Lynch, D.A.; Maher, T.M.; Martinez, F.J.; et al. Idiopathic Pulmonary Fibrosis (an Update) and Progressive Pulmonary Fibrosis in Adults: An Official ATS/ERS/JRS/ALAT Clinical Practice Guideline. *Am. J. Respir. Crit. Care Med.* **2022**, *205*, e18–e47. [CrossRef] [PubMed]
2. Recovery Collaborative Group; Horby, P.; Lim, W.S.; Emberson, J.R.; Mafham, M.; Bell, J.L.; Linsell, L.; Staplin, N.; Brightling, C.; Ustianowski, A.; et al. Dexamethasone in Hospitalized Patients with Covid-19. *N. Engl. J. Med.* **2021**, *384*, 693–704. [CrossRef] [PubMed]
3. Meyer, K.C. Immunosuppressive agents and interstitial lung disease: What are the risks? *Expert. Rev. Respir. Med.* **2014**, *8*, 263–266. [CrossRef] [PubMed]
4. Kondoh, Y.; Kataoka, K.; Ando, M.; Awaya, Y.; Ichikado, K.; Kataoka, M.; Komase, Y.; Mineshita, M.; Ohno, Y.; Okamoto, H.; et al. COVID-19 and acute exacerbation of interstitial lung disease. *Respir. Investig.* **2021**, *59*, 675–678. [CrossRef] [PubMed]
5. Gerver, S.M.; Guy, R.; Wilson, K.; Thelwall, S.; Nsonwu, O.; Rooney, G.; Brown, C.S.; Muller-Pebody, B.; Hope, R.; Hal, V. National surveillance of bacterial and fungal coinfection and secondary infection in COVID-19 patients in England: Lessons from the first wave. *Clin. Microbiol. Infect.* **2021**, *27*, 1658–1665. [CrossRef] [PubMed]
6. Garcia-Vidal, C.; Sanjuan, G.; Moreno-García, E.; Puerta-Alcalde, P.; Garcia-Pouton, N.; Chumbita, M.; Fernandez-Pittol, M.; Pitart, C.; Inciarte, A.; Bodro, M.; et al. Incidence of co-infections and superinfections in hospitalized patients with COVID-19: A retrospective cohort study. *Clin. Microbiol. Infect.* **2021**, *27*, 83–88. [CrossRef] [PubMed]
7. Youngs, J.; Wyncoll, D.; Hopkins, P.; Arnold, A.; Ball, J.; Bicanic, T. Improving antibiotic stewardship in COVID-19: Bacterial co-infection is less common than with influenza. *J. Infect.* **2020**, *81*, e55–e57. [CrossRef] [PubMed]
8. Ng, B.H.; Ban, A.Y.; Nik Abeed, N.N.; Faisal, M. Organising pneumonia manifesting as a late-phase complication of COVID-19. *BMJ Case Rep.* **2021**, *14*, e246119. [CrossRef] [PubMed]
9. Gentile, I.; Viceconte, G.; Lanzardo, A.; Zotta, I.; Zappulo, E.; Pinchera, B.; Scotto, R.; Schiano Moriello, N.; Foggia, M.; Giaccone, A.; et al. *Pneumocystis jirovecii* Pneumonia in Non-HIV Patients Recovering from COVID-19: A Single-Center Experience. *Int. J. Environ. Res. Public Health* **2021**, *18*, 11399. [CrossRef] [PubMed]
10. Fonte, L.; Acosta, A.; Sarmiento, M.E.; Norazmi, M.N.; Ginori, M.; de Armas, Y.; Calderón, E.J. Overlapping of Pulmonary Fibrosis of Postacute COVID-19 Syndrome and Tuberculosis in the Helminth Coinfection Setting in Sub-Saharan Africa. *Trop. Med. Infect. Dis.* **2022**, *7*, 157. [CrossRef]
11. Zhong-Jie, H.; Jia, X.; Ji-Ming, Y.; Li, L.; Wei, H.; Li-Li, Z.; Zhen, Z.; Yi-Zhou, Y.; Hong-Jun, L.; Ying-Mei, F.; et al. Lower Circulating Interferon-Gamma Is a Risk Factor for Lung Fibrosis in COVID-19 Patients. *Front. Immunol.* **2020**, *11*, 585647. [CrossRef]

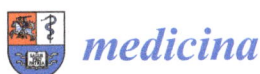

Case Report

Massive Spontaneous Pneumomediastinum—A Form of Presentation for Severe COVID-19 Pneumonia

Camelia Corina Pescaru [1,2], Monica Steluța Marc [1,2,*], Emanuela Oana Costin [1], Andrei Pescaru [3], Ana-Adriana Trusculescu [1,2], Adelina Maritescu [1,2], Noemi Suppini [1,2] and Cristian Iulian Oancea [1,2]

1. Pulmonology Department, 'Victor Babes' University of Medicine and Pharmacy, 300041 Timisoara, Romania
2. Center for Research and Innovation in Precision Medicine of Respiratory Diseases (CRIPMRD), 'Victor Babes' University of Medicine and Pharmacy, 300041 Timisoara, Romania
3. 'Victor Babes' University of Medicine and Pharmacy, 300041 Timisoara, Romania
* Correspondence: marc.monica@umft.ro

Abstract: For COVID-19 pneumonia, many manifestations such as fever, dyspnea, dry cough, anosmia and tiredness have been described, but differences have been observed from person to person according to age, pulmonary function, damage and severity. In clinical practice, it has been found that patients with severe forms of infection with COVID-19 develop serious complications, including pneumomediastinum. Although two years have passed since the beginning of the pandemic with the SARS-CoV-2 virus and progress has been made in understanding the pathophysiological mechanisms underlying the COVID-19 infection, there are also unknown factors that contribute to the evolution of the disease and can lead to the emergence some complications. In this case report, we present a patient with COVID-19 infection who developed a massive spontaneous pneumomediastinum and subcutaneous emphysema during hospitalization, with no pre-existing lung pathology and no history of smoking. The patient did not get mechanical ventilation or chest trauma, but the possible cause could be severe alveolar inflammation. The CT results highlighted pneumonia in context with SARS-CoV-2 infection affecting about 50% of the pulmonary area. During hospitalization, lung lesions evolved 80% pulmonary damage associated with pneumomediastinum and subcutaneous emphysema. After three months, the patient completely recovered and the pneumomediastinum fully recovered with the complete disappearance of the lesions. Pneumomediastinum is a severe and rare complication in COVID-19 pneumonia, especially in male patients, without risk factors, and an early diagnosis can increase the chances of survival.

Keywords: COVID-19; SARS-CoV-2; spontaneous pneumomediastinum; subcutaneous emphysema

Citation: Pescaru, C.C.; Marc, M.S.; Costin, E.O.; Pescaru, A.; Trusculescu, A.-A.; Maritescu, A.; Suppini, N.; Oancea, C.I. Massive Spontaneous Pneumomediastinum—A Form of Presentation for Severe COVID-19 Pneumonia. *Medicina* 2022, 58, 1525. https://doi.org/10.3390/medicina58111525

Academic Editor: Masaki Okamoto

Received: 29 September 2022
Accepted: 24 October 2022
Published: 26 October 2022

Publisher's Note: MDPI stays neutral with regard to jurisdictional claims in published maps and institutional affiliations.

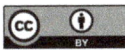

Copyright: © 2022 by the authors. Licensee MDPI, Basel, Switzerland. This article is an open access article distributed under the terms and conditions of the Creative Commons Attribution (CC BY) license (https://creativecommons.org/licenses/by/4.0/).

1. Introduction

Pneumomediastinum is a rare condition that represents the presence of air in the mediastinum. It is divided into two distinct types: spontaneous or secondary. Spontaneous pneumomediastinum is usually a self-condition, but it may be caused by precipitating factors such as: increased effort, recreational drugs, cough, vomiting effort, labor or Valsalva maneuvers [1].

Secondary pneumomediastinum is caused by a traumatic or damage to the mediastinum. It usually refers to an external factor such as chest injury, surgical complications, chronic lung disease, barotrauma or mechanical ventilation [2].

This condition generally occurs in young adults, especially in men [1]. The increased frequency in youth is due to the fact that their mediastinal tissue is loose, compared to the elders, whose tissues become fibrous with age. Thus, air can penetrate loose tissue much more easily than fibrous tissue [3].

Pneumomediastinum is a rare complication of COVID-19 pneumonia with an unknown mechanism, which is probably related to the increased alveolar pressure and pulmonary damage in people who develop severe forms of coronavirus disease [4]. This condition is based on the Macklin effect, which represents the alveolar rupture and air passage through the mediastinum due to increased thoracic pressure and severe inflammation [5].

The incidence of pneumomediastinum in COVID-19 pneumonia in patients without lung history disease is around 16.6%, as proved by an Iranian study [6].

Although it is considered a rare phenomenon, the prevalence of pneumomediastinum in COVID-19 pneumomia has been continually increasing in comparison with patients with adult respiratory distress syndrome since 2003, when it was 4%. This could be happened because of the compressed air injury, level of barotrauma and higher susceptibility in the population infected with SARS-CoV-2; it was also observed that men are more likely to develop the problem [7].

The novelty of this case report consists in the fact that a young patient without comorbidities except OSAS developed massive pneumomediastinum, including subcutaneous emphysema, for which the patient was monitored long-term and completely recovered 3 months after the onset.

In the clinical trial, the most common symptoms were chest pain with irradiation to the neck or back, unexplained and unexpected dyspnea and subcutaneous emphysema. It may include other symptoms such as cough, neck pain, or vomiting, or it could be asymptomatic. It is a life-threatening condition that must be carefully monitored [8,9].

2. Materials and Methods

Case Presentation

A 45-year-old man with a history of essential hypertension and sleep apnea, both under treatment, came to the hospital presenting the following symptoms: a high-grade fever of 39 °C, shortness of breath, muscle pain, fatigue and anosmia. Blood pressure was 145/82 mmHg, the pulse was 95 bpm, his respiratory rate was 35 and oxygen saturation was 91% on room air. The real-time reverse transcription-polymerase chain reaction (RT-PCR) for SARS-CoV-2 was positive, but the patient refused hospitalization and went home with a treatment scheme based on symptomatics, vitamins and antibiotics. After 3 days, his grade of fever increased, his condition had depreciated and he decided to come back for investigations. Laboratory tests showed that the level of C-reactive protein, ferritin, LDH, D-dimers, were elevated, and the patient also had moderate hepatocytolysis and a high level of blood glucose (Table 1).

Table 1. Complete blood count.

Laboratory Test	Conventional Units	Value	Reference Range Value
WBC	$*10^3/\mu L$	5.05	4.00–10.00
Lymphocytes	$*10^3/\mu L$	0.74	1.20–4.40
Monocyte	$*10^3/\mu L$	0.6	0.22–1.00
Interleukin 6	Pg/mL	50.75	<9.7
LDH	U/L	778	135–225
Blood glucose	mg/dL	126	74–106
Ferritin	µg/L	2861.6	30–400
D-dimers	µg/mL	0.62	<0.5
AST	U/L	226.1	0–40
ALT	U/L	124.8	0–41
CRP	mg/L	79.9	0–5
aPTT	seconds	25.4	25–36
PCR Covid	positive/negative	positive	-

* WBC, white blood cells; LDH, lactate dehydrogenase; AST, aspartate aminotransferase; ALT, alanine aminotransferase; CRP–C, reactive protein; aPTT, active partial thromboplastin time.

The initial CT results presented the appearance of pneumonia in the context of SARS-CoV-2 infection (moderate form), affecting approximately 50% of the lung area. He started treatment with antivirals in the first stage; corticosteroids, vitamins and anticoagulants according to guidelines. The patient benefited from antiviral therapy with Favipiravir—200 mg/tablet; on the first day 16 tablets (8–0–8), then 8 tablets/day (4–0–4) for 7 days; Anakinra—150 mg/mL, 4 syringes/ on the first day (2–0–2) then 1/day; Corticotherapy—Dexamethasone vial of 8 mg, 2 × 1/ day for 10 days; anticoagulant Fraxiparine 8600 iu/0.8 mL, once a day throughout the hospitalization period for prophylactic purposes; Pantoprazole 40 mg bottle, 2/day, for 10 days; ascorbic acid vial of 750 mg, 2/day, codeine 15 mg, 2 tablets/day; and oxygenoterapy 10 L/min through the reservoir mask, maintaining oxygen saturation over 94%. He remained on oxygen therapy, vitamins and antitussives for the entire hospitalization period.

The patient presented severe OSAS, but with hemodynamic stability and relatively well-tolerated daytime and nighttime symptoms, which correlated with the patient's current situation, required the timing of the administration of nighttime treatment with CPAP-type continuous positive air pressure. This timing was taken into account precisely to prevent this air leak syndrome (pneumothorax with bronchopleural fistula). Compliance with hygiene–dietary rules with weight loss and nutritional counseling plus compliance with sleep hygiene rules were recommended.

During the hospitalization, on day 14, the patient presented coughing, dyspnea, retrosternal pain and crackles were noted around his neck and chest area; symptoms suggestive of pneumomediastinum and subcutaneous emphysema. A CT was performed and confirmed severe pneumomediastinum with extensive subcutaneous emphysema (Figure 1); the lung damage had increased to 80%. The thoracic surgeon team considered it better to wait before a surgical approach, mainly because a spontaneous pneumomediastinum is very probable to absorb by itself. After three days of continuous monitoring, the status of the patient gradually improved. He was included in respiratory rehabilitation programs due to his fatigue and difficulty in breathing, and the clinical status of the patient was improved. The subcutaneous emphysema disappeared with superficial palpation and his oxygen saturation improved to 95% on room air. Because of the respiratory rehabilitation exercises, the patient overcame his fear of breathing again and of making a minimum breathing effort (things he forgot during the illness). This improvement helped to reduce his anxiety and mental state. His recovery was almost completed, being discharged from hospital after 30 days in a stable condition. Three months later, the reassessment CT showed that pneumomediastinum and emphysema were completely absorbed (Figure 1).

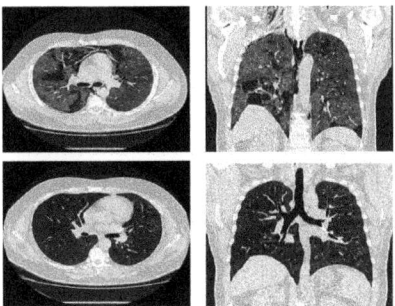

Figure 1. Thoracic CT showing pneumomediastinum and CT, three-months later, showing complete remission of pneumomediastinum.

3. Discussion

The development of spontaneous pneumomediastinum is a challenging complication for healthcare workers in patients with SARS-CoV2 infection. It can be spontaneous or secondary and represents a gaseous infiltration into mediastinal cellular tissues.

Although pneumomediastinum occurs most recently in COVID-19 pneumonia, the main causes of its occurrence remain the ones mentioned above. The factors that may increase the risk of developing this condition are smoking, male sex, age, asthma, COPD or symptoms such as prolonged cough and excessive vomiting. Subcutaneous crepitations occur when air gets into the tissues under the skin and represents the appearance of subcutaneous emphysema, a major sign of pneumomediastinum [10]. Radiology is fundamental in diagnostic pneumomediastin, X-ray being the first intent investigation. However, thorax CT is used to diagnose pneumomediastinum in situations where X-ray is not sufficient, and can provide additional information about pre-existing parenchymal or pleural pulmonary pathologies. Guidelines recommend having an X-ray for young patients who present unexplained dyspnea and chest pain [11].

We concluded that our patient developed spontaneous pneumomediastinum because of the severe injuries caused by COVID-19 infection, considering the fact that he did not have risk factors. The most probable mechanism of producing it was based on the Macklin effect, the alveolar rupture and air passage through the mediastinum, due to increased intrathoracic pressure and important inflammation [8]. The patient suddenly presented dyspnoea, chest pain, hypoxia and tachycardia, so a native thoracic CT scan was performed in order to exclude other differential diagnoses, such as pulmonary embolism. The normal value of D-dimers biologically ruled out the diagnosis of pulmonary thromboembolism in the dynamics throughout the hospitalization, and pneumothorax was ruled out by pulmonary CT.

The CT scan confirmed a huge pneumomediastinum, which challenged the medical team to consider therapeutic management for this interesting case, with such a complication of SARS-CoV-2 infection. Although the diagnosis was established, it was better to wait than take action. Therefore, in this case, it was preferred to provide vital functions and simple therapeutic measures, such as oxygen and analgesics, with a good outcome. Due to prompt radiological investigations in our hospital, patients with COVID-19 benefited from rapid diagnosis and correct evaluation of lung lesions, thus being able to provide adequate treatment and prompt management. This case was a successful one; the patient had a favorable evolution so that he was discharged with a good general condition, and at the control thoracic CT scan at 3 months, both the lung lesions and the pneumomediastinum were returned.

Although two years have passed since the beginning of the pandemic with the SARS-CoV-2 virus and progress has been made in understanding the pathophysiological mechanisms underlying the COVID-19 infection, there are also unknown factors that contribute to the evolution of the disease and can lead to the emergence of severe complications [12].

Anxiety is often present, but in patients who develop pneumomediastinum as a complication, the level of anxiety is increased and requires treatment [1]. Physical examination reveals crepitus at palpation when there is subcutaneous emphysema involved [13]. A sound like bursting balloons is frequently detected by the patient. The Hamman sign is pathognomic for mediastinal emphysema and represents a synchronous sound with the heartbeat, specifically produced by the difference of the heartbeat against air-filled tissues in the left precordial border [14]. The standard diagnosis is made by chest radiography or chest CT when an X-ray is inconclusive. The differential diagnosis should be made with conditions that present symptoms such as dyspnea, chest pain and hypoxia, so taking into consideration pulmonary embolism, pneumothorax, coronary syndrome or pericarditis is always necessary. Complications are rare, but if hypertensive pneumomendiastinum is involved, vessel compression could affect the venous blood return and this may compromise the hemodynamic and respiratory system. On the other hand, mediastinitis are also a serious complication, but the mortality, in this case, is increased by the coexisting illnesses [1]. Developing pneumomediastinum in this viral infection may be an indicator of worsening disease, but our patient luckily survived due to the proper investigations, diagnosis and suitable management, and his status was completely recovered [15].

4. Conclusions

In conclusion, pneumomediastinum in COVID-19 can also occur in young patients without pre-existing lung pathology with the exception of OSAS in this case but with acute respiratory distress syndrome which may represent the physiopathological production mechanism for pneumoemdiastinum. Although pneumomediastinum is a very rare complication in the evolution of the COVID-19 infection, it can be life-threatening for the patient. In the presented case, the evolution was favorable, with complete resorption of the pneumomediastinum within 3 months of the occurrence.

Author Contributions: Conceptualization, C.C.P., M.S.M. and A.-A.T.; methodology, C.C.P. and A.M.; validation, C.C.P. and M.S.M.; formal analysis, C.C.P. and A.M.; investigation, C.C.P., M.S.M., N.S. and E.O.C.; resources, C.I.O. and M.S.M.; data curation, E.O.C., A.P. and N.S.; writing—original draft preparation, C.C.P., A.M. and E.O.C.; writing—review and editing, C.C.P. and A.-A.T.; supervision, C.I.O. and A.-A.T.; project administration, C.I.O. All authors have read and agreed to the published version of the manuscript.

Funding: This research received no external funding.

Institutional Review Board Statement: The study was conducted in accordance with the Declaration of Helsinki: and approved by the Ethics Committee of Clinical Hospital for Infectious Diseases and Pneumoftiziology Victor Babeș Timișoara for studies involving humans.

Informed Consent Statement: Informed consent was obtained from all subjects involved in the study.

Data Availability Statement: The data presented in this study are available on reasonable request from the corresponding author.

Conflicts of Interest: The authors declare no conflict of interest.

References

1. Meireles, J.; Neves, S.; Castro, A.; França, M. Spontaneous pneumomediastinum revisited. *Respir. Med. CME* **2011**, *4*, 181–183. [CrossRef]
2. Marza, A.M.; Petrica, A.; Buleu, F.N.; Mederle, O.A. Case report: Massive spontaneous pneumothorax—A rare form of presentation for severe COVID-19 pneumonia. *Medicina* **2021**, *57*, 82. [CrossRef] [PubMed]
3. Alemu, B.N.; Yeheyis, E.T.; Tiruneh, A.G. Spontaneous primary pneumomediastinum: Is it always benign? *J. Med. Case Rep.* **2021**, *15*, 157. [CrossRef] [PubMed]
4. Loffi, M.; Regazzoni, V.; Sergio, P.; Martinelli, E.; Stifani, I.; Quinzani, F.; Robba, D.; Cotugno, A.; Dede, M.; Danzi, G.B. Spontaneous pneumomediastinum in COVID-19 pneumonia. *Monaldi Arch. Chest Dis.* **2020**. [CrossRef] [PubMed]
5. Macklin, M.T.; Macklin, C.C. Malignant interstitial emphysema of the lungs and mediastinum as an important occult complication in many respiratory diseases and other conditions: An interpretation of the clinical literature in the light of laboratory experiment. *Medicine* **1944**, *23*, 281–358. [CrossRef]
6. Underner, M.; Peiffer, G.; Perriot, J.; Jaafari, N. Spontaneous pneumomediastinum: A rare complication of COVID-19? *Rev. Des. Mal. Respir.* **2020**, *37*, 680–683. [CrossRef] [PubMed]
7. Kangas-Dick, A.; Gazivoda, V.; Ibrahim, M.; Sun, A.; Shaw, J.P.; Brichkov, I.; Wiesel, O. Clinical Characteristics and Outcome of Pneumomediastinum in Patients with COVID-19 Pneumonia. *J. Laparoendosc. Adv. Surg. Tech. A* **2021**, *31*, 273–278. [CrossRef] [PubMed]
8. Kong, N.; Gao, C.; Xu, M.S.; Xie, Y.L.; Zhou, C.Y. Spontaneous pneumomediastinum in an elderly COVID-19 patient: A case report. *World J. Clin. Cases* **2020**, *8*, 3573–3577. [CrossRef] [PubMed]
9. Kara, H.; Uyar, H.G.; Degirmenci, S.; Bayir, A.; Oncel, M.; Ak, A. Dyspnoea and chest pain as the presenting symptoms of pneumomediastinum: Two cases and a review of the literature. *Cardiovasc. J. Afr.* **2015**, *26*, 1–4. [CrossRef] [PubMed]
10. Janssen, J.; Kamps, M.J.A.; Joosten, T.M.B.; Barten, D.G. Spontaneous pneumomediastinum in a male adult with COVID-19 pneumonia. *Am. J. Emerg. Med.* **2021**. [CrossRef] [PubMed]
11. Mobarek, S.K. Persistent unexplained chest pain and dyspnea in a patient with coronary artery disease: A case report. *BMC Cardiovasc. Disord.* **2020**. [CrossRef] [PubMed]
12. Pescaru, C.C.; Marițescu, A.; Costin, E.O.; Trăilă, D.; Marc, M.S.; Trușculescu, A.A.; Pescaru, A.; Oancea, C.I. The Effects of COVID-19 on Skeletal Muscles, Muscle Fatigue and Rehabilitation Programs Outcomes. *Medicina (Kaunas)* **2022**, *58*, 1199. [CrossRef] [PubMed]
13. Dirweesh, A.; Alvarez, C.; Khan, M.; Christmas, D. Spontaneous pneumomediastinum in a healthy young female: A case report and literature review. *Respir. Med. Case Rep.* **2017**, *20*, 129–132. [CrossRef] [PubMed]

14. Kelly, S.; Hughes, S.; Nixon, S.; Paterson-Brown, S. Spontaneous pneumomediastinum (Hamman's syndrome). *Surgeon* **2010**, *8*, 63–66. [CrossRef]
15. Elhakim, T.S.; Abdul, H.S.; Pelaez Romero, C.; Rodriguez-Fuentes, Y. Spontaneous pneumomediastinum, pneumothorax and subcutaneous emphysema in COVID-19 pneumonia: A rare case and literature review. *BMJ Case Rep.* **2020**, *13*, e239489. [CrossRef]

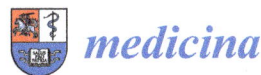

Article

Efficacy of Therapeutic Plasma Exchange in Severe Acute Respiratory Distress Syndrome in COVID-19 Patients from the Western Part of Romania

Tamara Mirela Porosnicu [1,†], Ciprian Gindac [2,*,†], Sonia Popovici [2], Adelina Marinescu [3], Daniel Jipa [2], Valentina Lazaroiu [4], Dorel Sandesc [5], Cristian Oancea [6], Roxana Folescu [7,*], Alexandra-Simona Zamfir [8], Carmen Lacramioara Zamfir [9,*], Laura Alexandra Nussbaum [10] and Ioan Ovidiu Sirbu [1]

1. Center for Complex Network Science "V.Babes", University of Medicine and Pharmacy, 2 Eftimie Murgu Sq., 300041 Timisoara, Romania
2. Intensive Care Unit "Pius Branzeu", Emergency Clinical County Hospital, Liviu Rebreanu 156, 300723 Timisoara, Romania
3. Discipline of Infectious Diseases, Department XIII, "V.Babes" University of Medicine and Pharmacy, 2 Eftimie Murgu Sq., 300041 Timisoara, Romania
4. Clinical Hospital of Infectious Diseases and Pneumo Phtisiology "Doctor V.Babes", Gh.Adam 13 Street, 300310 Timisoara, Romania
5. Department of Anaesthesia and Intensive Care "V.Babes" University of Medicine and Pharmacy, 2 Eftimie Murgu Sq., 300041 Timisoara, Romania
6. Center for Research and Innovation in Personalized Respiratory Disease Medicine, "V.Babes" University of Medicine and Pharmacy, 2 Eftimie Murgu Sq., 300041 Timisoara, Romania
7. Department of Balneology, Medical Recovery and Rheumatology, Family Medicine Discipline, Center for Preventive Medicine for Advanced Research in Cardiovascular Pathology and Hemostaseology, "V.Babes" University of Medicine and Pharmacy, 2 Eftimie Murgu Sq., 300041 Timisoara, Romania
8. Department of Internal Medicine III, Discipline of Pneumology, "Grigore T. Popa" University of Medicine and Pharmacy, 16 University Str., 700115 Iasi, Romania
9. Department of Morpho-Functional Sciences I, "Grigore T. Popa" University of Medicine and Pharmacy, 16 University Str., 700115 Iasi, Romania
10. Department of Neurosciences, "V.Babes" University of Medicine and Pharmacy, 2 Eftimie Murgu Sq., 300041 Timisoara, Romania
* Correspondence: ciprian.gindac@gmail.com (C.G.); folescu.roxana@umft.ro (R.F.); carmen.zamfir@umfiasi.ro (C.L.Z.)
† These authors contributed equally to this work.

Abstract: *Background and Objectives*: The COVID-19 pandemic, caused by the SARS-CoV-2 virus, has surprised the medical world with its devastating effects such as severe acute respiratory distress syndrome (ARDS) and cytokine storm, but also with the scant therapeutic solutions which have proven to be effective against the disease. Therapeutic plasma exchange (TPE) has been proposed from the very beginning as a possible adjuvant treatment in severe cases. Our objective was to analyze the evolution of specific biological markers of the COVID-19 disease before and one day after a therapeutic plasma exchange session, how a change in these parameters influences the patient's respiratory status, as well as the impact of TPE on the survival rate. *Materials and Methods*: In this retrospective study, we include 65 patients with COVID-19 admitted to the intensive care unit department of our hospital between March 2020 and December 2021, and who received a total of 120 sessions of TPE. *Results*: TPE significantly reduced the following inflammation markers ($p < 0.001$): interleukin-6 (IL-6), C-reactive protein (CRP), lactate dehydrogenase (LDH), fibrinogen, ferritin, and erythrocyte sedimentation rate. This procedure significantly increased the number of lymphocytes and decreased D-dimers levels ($p = 0.0024$). TPE significantly improved the PaO_2/FiO_2 ratio ($p < 0.001$) in patients with severe acute respiratory distress syndrome ($PaO_2/FiO_2 < 100$). Survival was improved in intubated patients who received TPE. *Conclusions*: TPE involved the reduction in inflammatory markers in critical patients with COVID-19 disease and the improvement of the PaO_2/FiO_2 ratio in patients with severe ARDS and had a potential benefit on the survival of patients with extremely severe COVID-19 disease.

Citation: Porosnicu, T.M.; Gindac, C.; Popovici, S.; Marinescu, A.; Jipa, D.; Lazaroiu, V.; Sandesc, D.; Oancea, C.; Folescu, R.; Zamfir, A.-S.; et al. Efficacy of Therapeutic Plasma Exchange in Severe Acute Respiratory Distress Syndrome in COVID-19 Patients from the Western Part of Romania. *Medicina* 2022, 58, 1707. https://doi.org/10.3390/medicina58121707

Academic Editor: Masaki Okamoto

Received: 31 October 2022
Accepted: 20 November 2022
Published: 23 November 2022

Publisher's Note: MDPI stays neutral with regard to jurisdictional claims in published maps and institutional affiliations.

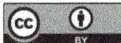

Copyright: © 2022 by the authors. Licensee MDPI, Basel, Switzerland. This article is an open access article distributed under the terms and conditions of the Creative Commons Attribution (CC BY) license (https:// creativecommons.org/licenses/by/ 4.0/).

Keywords: therapeutic plasma exchange; ARDS; inflammatory markers; COVID-19; survival

1. Introduction

The COVID-19 pandemic, caused by the SARS-CoV-2 virus, has surprised the entire medical world with its devastating effects of severe ARDS [1] and cytokine storm [2], but also by the scant therapeutic solutions which have proven to be effective against the disease. A number of antivirals, [3,4] immunomodulatory [5–7], corticosteroid [8], and anticoagulant therapies [9] have aroused interest in treating patients with COVID-19 disease who require intensive therapy, with or without mechanical ventilation. Among the plasma purification techniques, therapeutic plasma exchange (TPE) has been proposed from the very beginning as a possible adjuvant treatment in severe cases requiring admission to intensive care [10]. The rationale behind using TPE for the treatment of COVID-19 patients includes the reduction in inflammatory cytokines levels, the stabilization of the endothelial membrane, treatment of hyperviscosity, reduction in antifibrinolytic mediators, and fibrin degradation products or the elimination of SARS-CoV-2 virus [11]. Therapeutic plasma exchange can eliminate the mediators excessively released in the cytokine storm and improve the biomarkers related to a poor prognosis. These are large molecules (IL-6 = 28 kDa, ferritin = 475 kDa, LDH = 140 kDa, CRP = 25 kDa, D-dimers = 180 kDa, fibrinogen = 340kDa) that can be eliminated by a plasma-filter [12].

The main purpose of this study was to analyze the evolution of specific biological markers in COVID-19 disease before and one day after a TPE session and how the change in these parameters influences the patient's respiratory status, as well as the impact of TPE on survival rates. All the patients received antiviral, anticoagulant, and corticosteroid treatment.

2. Materials and Methods

2.1. Experimental Part

Study period: Between March 2020 and December 2021, more than 4500 patients from the western part of Romania who were infected with the SARS-CoV-2 virus were treated in our hospital. The Clinical Hospital of Infectious Diseases and Pneumo-Phthisiology "Doctor V.Babes", Timisoara, was the main hospital that treated patients with COVID-19 in the western part of Romania. During this period, 535 patients were admitted to the intensive care unit (ICU) with severe forms of the disease, out of which over 401 patients required intubation and mechanical ventilation. Patients admitted to the ICU during this period presented severe lung damage (moderate or severe ARDS). Therapeutic plasma exchange was initiated in 65 adult patients who experienced a severe impairment of respiratory status or an increase in specific biological markers (IL-6, ferritin, ESR, D-dimers, LDH, CRP, and fibrinogen) for excessive cytokine release syndrome as a complication of COVID-19.

Ethical aspects: The study was conducted in the ICU department and the written informed consent was obtained from all study participants. The Ethical Committee of the hospital (nr. 13037/24/12/2021) approved the study.

Inclusion criteria in patient selection were that patients were aged over 18 years, had moderate or severe ARDS and/or cytokine storm (exaggerated increase in specific parameters for systemic inflammation), in addition to the availability of clinical and laboratory data before and at one day after conducting TPE sessions. Our patients had clinical respiratory deterioration requiring admission to the intensive care unit and needed increased oxygen (more than 30 L/min), $SpO_2 < 90\%$, respiratory rate over 30 breaths/min, and $PaO_2/FiO_2 < 200$ mmHg (moderate ARDS $100 \leq PaO_2/FiO_2 < 200$ or severe ARDS = $PaO_2/FiO_2 < 100$).

Data collection: A series of demographic data were analyzed: age, sex, BMI, respiratory status, number of days from the beginning of COVID-19 symptoms until the first TPE, number of sessions of TPE, and comorbidities (diabetes, hypertension, obesity, and COPD).

Variables: The following parameters were included for the analysis: biological markers for inflammation (IL-6, CRP, ferritin, D-dimers, ESR, LDH, procalcitonin, and fibrinogen). Leukocyte count, lymphocytes count and percentage, hemodynamic parameters, vasopressor requirement, and temperature were also analyzed.

To evaluate the impact of organ failure after the TPE session, we investigated liver enzymes, blood urea nitrogen (BUN), creatinine, pH, lactate, SOFA, and APACHE II scores. Oxygenated status of the patients was examined using the following: PaO_2/FiO_2, respiratory rate, ROXINDEX score, HACOR score, and the oxygenation index (OI).

The TPE sessions were performed using the Prismaflex (Baxter International, Deerfield, IL, USA) device with a TPE 2000 plasma-filter or by using the HF404 machine (Infomed) with a Granopen 60 plasma-filter (LF 060-00). As a substitute, 5% human albumin solution or fresh frozen plasma were used in doses of 1–1.3 times the patient's plasma volume. Fractionated heparin and/or citrate were used as an anticoagulant [13]. We did not use convalescent plasma for these patients.

The determination of biochemical parameters was performed at a hospital laboratory with the COBAS INTEGRA 400 plus device (Roche diagnostics) and the reverse transcription polymerase chain reaction (RT-PCR) for SARS-CoV-2 with a BIONEER extractor and EXICYCLER 96 amplifier (Bioneer, Daejeon, Republic of Korea). COVID-19 case confirmation was obtained using the CFX96 Real-Time PCR Systems (Bio-Rad, Hercules, CA, USA). The viral RNA was extracted with the NIMBUS extractor, using the STARMag 96X4 Universal Cartridge Kit (Seegene, Seoul, Republic of Korea).

2.2. Statistical Analysis

A data analysis was performed using the Statistical Package for Social Sciences v.25 (IBM SPSS Statistics, Chicago, IL, USA). A p value of less than 0.05 was considered statistically significant. Paired sample Wilcoxon tests were used for the statistical analysis. Due to the small sample size of the data set, we prefer this test for our data. There were a few huge values for some covariates (such as IL6 over 5000 pg/mL), which is why Wilcoxon's test may be more appropriate. Quantitative variables were tested for normal distribution and compared by means of a Wilcoxon test paired sample.

3. Results

We analyzed data from 65 adult patients and 120 TPE procedures: 41 patients with 1 session, 13 patients with 2 sessions, and 11 patients with 3 or more sessions (2 with 3 sessions, 4 with 4 sessions, 1 with 5 sessions, 2 with 6 sessions, and 2 with 7 sessions) (Table 1).

Table 1. Demographic and baseline characteristics of critical patients with COVID-19 (n = 65).

Age-mean (min–max)	52.70 (21–80)
Body Mass Index-mean	33.2
Gender	
Male	45
Female	20
Days from RT-PCR COVID-19 and TPE mean, (min–max)	16.6 (5–51)
Respiratory status	
Invasive Mechanical Ventilation	40
Noninvasive Mechanical Ventilation	25

Table 1. *Cont.*

Comorbidities (no. and % from total no. of patients)	
Diabetes Mellitus	10 (15.38%)
Hypertension	33 (50.76%)
Obesity	27 (41.53%)
COPD/asthma	6 (9.23%)
No. of sessions (total)	120
Patients with 1 session	41
Patients with 2 sessions	13
Patients with more than 2 sessions	11

RT-PCR: reverse transcription polymerase chain reaction; COPD: chronic obstructive pulmonary disease.

Laboratory and clinical data of patients with COVID-19 were analyzed one day before and one day after TPE and using the Wilcoxon test paired sample (Table 2). These 65 patients had moderate or severe ARDS (PaO_2/FiO_2 median was 98.25) or an increased inflammatory marker [14].

Table 2. Average and medium values of analyzed biological markers, before and after TPE, *p*-value. (n = 65).

Variable	Average/Median before TPE	Average/Median after TPE	*p*-Value for Median
IL-6, pg/ml	799/129	480/79	0.0003
Ferritin, µg/L	2364/1529	1660/1120	<0.0001
D-dimers, µg/ml	5.18/1.9	3.50/1.57	0.0024
CRP, mg/L	122/88	87/60	0.0001
LDH, U/L	579/512	461/419	<0.0001
PCT, ng/ml	2.28/0.33	2.26/0.42	0.34
Fibrinogen, g/L	4.90/4.23	3.42/3.26	<0.0001
ESR, mm/h	46/35	22/15	<0.0001
Leucocytes, $\times 10^3/\mu L$	14/13	16/15.5	0.19
% Lymphocytes	7.66/5.2	8.14/5.5	0.53
Lymph abs, $\times 10^3/\mu L$	0.96/0.69	1.11/0.80	0.003
TAM, mmHg	80.9/77	81.9/80	0.9
Temperature, °C	36.5/36.4	36.6/36.4	0.26
BUN, mg/dL	72.7/58.5	74.2/62	0.29
Creatinine, mg/dL	1.02/0.8	1.08/0.81	0.98
PH	7.42/7.43	7.41/7.42	0.79
Lactate, mmol/L	2.49/2.30	2.55/2.27	0.72
SOFA	7.71/7	7.76/7	0.96
APACHE 2	11.7/11	12.1/12	0.056
PaO_2/FiO_2	128.1/98.25	131.7/113.25	0.23
P/F < 100 for 55 sessions	75/77	92/90	**0.0002**
P/F ≥ 100 for 55 sessions	184/168	173/162	0.17

IL-6: intrleukin-6; CRP-C reactive protein; LDH: lactate dehydrogenase; PCT: procalcitonin; ESR: erythrocyte sedimentation rate; TAM-mean arterial pressure; BUN: blood urea nitrogen; SOFA: Sequential Organ Failure assessment; APACHE 2: Acute Physiology and Chronic Health Evaluation; PaO_2/FiO_2: pressure of arterial oxygen to fractional inspired oxygen concentration; P/F: pressure of arterial oxygen to fractional inspired oxygen concentration; TPE: therapeutic plasma exchange.

A lot of covariates were analyzed before and after 120 TPE sessions for 65 patients. There were only 110 sessions to evaluate the PaO_2/FiO_2 ratio after TPE. We excluded data from 10 sessions for patients on ECMO (Table 1). This section may be divided by subheadings. It should provide a concise and precise description of the experimental results, their interpretation, as well as the experimental conclusions that can be drawn.

Large molecules such as ferritin, D-dimers, CRP (C-reactive protein), fibrinogen, LDH (lactate dehydrogenase), and IL-6 were eliminated by TPE in most of the cases with a strong statistical significance, as we expected ($p < 0.05$, Table 2). In our group, the average values for these markers before the first TPE session are: IL-6 = 799 pg/mL, ferritin = 2364 µg/L, D-dimers = 5.18 µg/mL, CRP = 122 mg/L, LDH = 579 U/L, and fibrinogen = 4.90 g/L) (Table 2).

There was no statistically significant improvement in the following studied clinical features: pulmonary status (respiratory rate, PaO_2/FiO_2, OI), hemodynamic parameters (TAM, AV, and need for vasopressor agents), organ functionality (BUN, creatinine, lactate, SOFA and APACHE II score), none of which were improved ($p > 0.5$). We observed that the median lymphocyte percentage or the absolute count improved after TPE procedure. A particular group with severe ARDS ($PaO_2/FiO_2 < 100$) had a statistically significant improvement in oxygenation after TPE ($p = 0.002$) (Figure 1). The rest of the patients with mild/moderate ARDS had no statistically significant improvement in oxygenation after TPE sessions ($p = 0.17$) (Figure 2). The mean value for PaO_2/FiO_2 in the group with severe ARDS increased from 75 to 92; the mean decreased from in the rest of the group 184 to 173 (Figures 1 and 2).

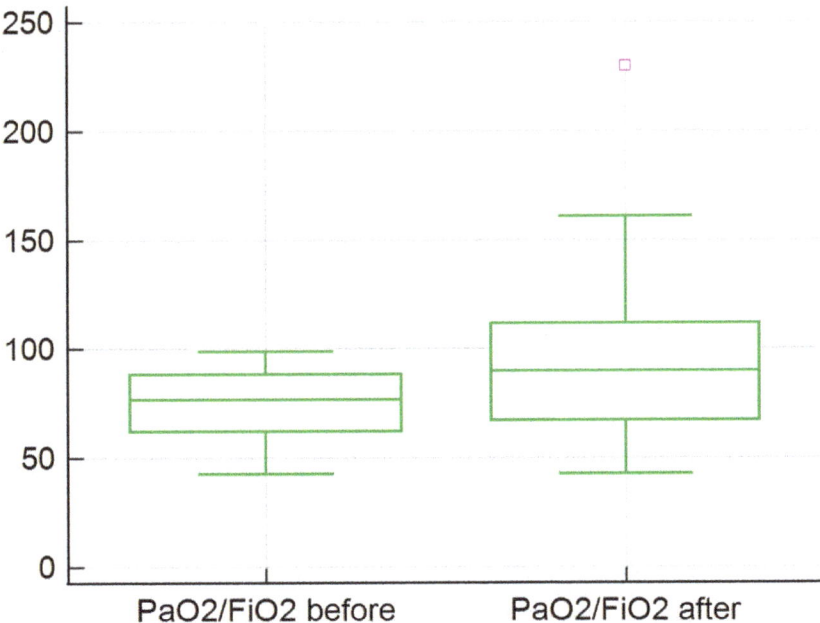

Figure 1. TPE impact on the PaO_2/FiO_2 ratio in patients with severe ARDS (55 sessions).

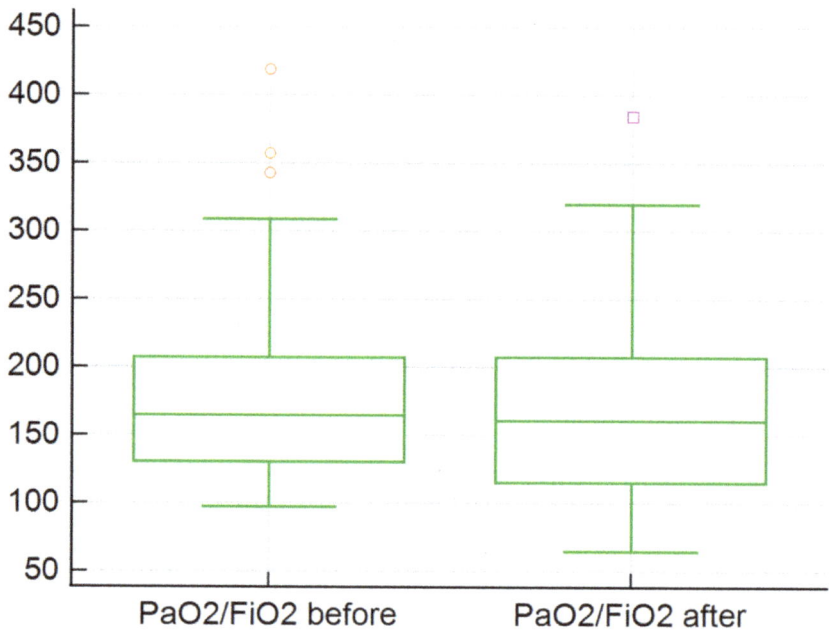

Figure 2. TPE impact on PaO_2/FiO_2 ratio in patients with non-severe ARDS (55 sessions).

A total of 61% of the patients included in the study were mechanically ventilated at the time of the first TPE. The oxygenation index (OI) was 21.56 before TPE and 21.8 after TPE and four patients needed ECMO (where the P/F ratio has no reason to be evaluated). There were only 16 survivors in our 65-patient group after 28 days (24.61%). Between 40 mechanical ventilated patients, there were 7 survivors. In the subgroup of 11 patients with more than 2 TPE procedures/patient (average 4.8), the P/F ratio remained at the same: the median value is 121 before TPE versus 122 after TPE, and an average of 144 versus 147. There was no statistically significant impact on the P/F ratio ($p = 0.36$). More than two TPE sessions for one patient had no statistically significant benefit in oxygenation in our study. In 63 of the TPE sessions, we have observed an improvement in P/F ratio, whereas in the other 47 sessions, no improvement after TPE was shown. In the group with severe ARDS in 55 TPE sessions, 41 resulted in an improvement in oxygenation and in the other group with moderate/mild ARDS in 55 sessions, only 22 had an improvement in oxygenation.

From a total number of 535 patients admitted to ICU, 401 were finally invasively mechanical ventilated, and 375 died and 160 survived. Only 26 from the intubated patients (6.5%) survived. From a total of 65 patients who performed TPE, 56 were invasively mechanical ventilated from the beginning; a total of 16 of them survived and 7 from the intubated patients (12.5%). There was an improvement in the survival rate ($p = 0.05$) between patients with invasive mechanical ventilation and who had TPE performed on them compared to the survival rate of the patients with invasive mechanical ventilation without TPE (5.2%) in our ICU department along this period of COVID-19 disease (Figure 3).

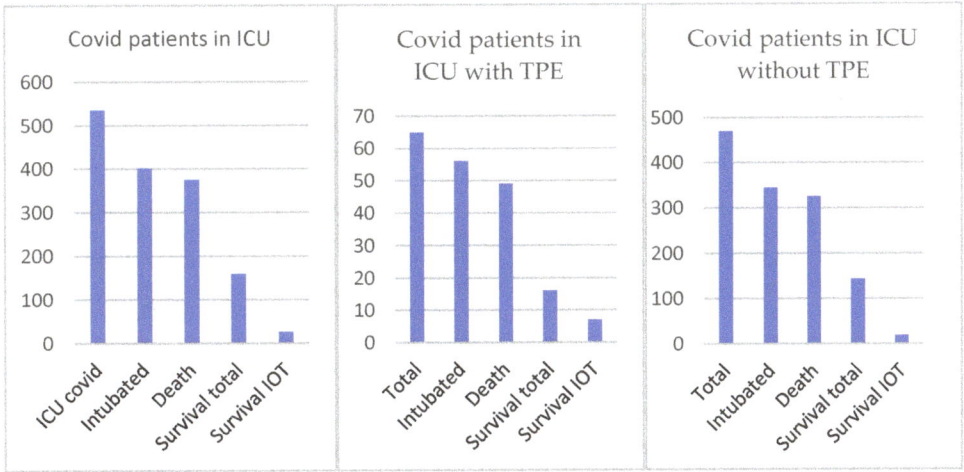

Figure 3. Survival in ICU: total COVID patients versus COVID patients with/without TPE.

4. Discussion

The SARS-CoV-2 virus had a global impact and there are still no clear treatments for moderate and severe ARDS in COVID-19 patients. More than 50% of patients with cytokine storm develop ARDS and early recognition and control of dysregulated immune response are essential [15].

Our study showed that TPE significantly reduced the levels of the main inflammatory biomarkers associated with a poor prognosis. Therapeutic plasma exchange had a positive impact on the respiratory status (improvement in PaO_2/FiO_2) in patients with a P/F ratio under 100. Moreover, we also observed slight improvements in patients with a P/F ratio over 100. The impact of TPE in the COVID-19 critically ill patient was not significant regarding the case of end-organ failure.

The first extrarenal clearance procedures were tried in patients with COVID-19 in Asia [16]. Case series and individual reports have shown the effectiveness of TPE in the reduction in inflammation markers [16]. The results seemed very encouraging and suggested both the overall reduction in inflammation markers and the improvement of respiratory parameters: reduction in oxygen demand, decrease in respiratory rate, and early extubating [16]. With the outbreak of the pandemic, it has been observed that there is a link between the severity of the disease following infection with the SARS-CoV-2 virus and a series of biological markers whose values are altered. Changes in these markers (IL-6, IL-1, TNFα, D-dimers, CRP, ferritin, LDH, and fibrinogen), especially inflammatory ones, have a specificity for a poor prognosis [17]. Subsequently, attempts were made to demonstrate the reduction in inflammation markers by a series of plasma purification procedures, by the administration of immunomodulatory agents, and with the use of anti-inflammatory drugs. Out of these options, TPE significantly reduced specific markers in the case of cytokine storm (CS) but had less impact on respiratory parameters or survival rate [18].

There have been few studies in the literature that have analyzed the data of patients receiving TPE and patients receiving only standard therapy [13,19,20]. Thus, Fahad Faqihi et al. [19], in a randomized study, analyzed 43 patients who received standard treatment plus TPE and 44 patients who received only standard treatment and observed that mortality at 35 days in the group who received TPE compared to the control group was not significantly lower (20.9% vs. 34.1%), *p*-value 0.58. However, biological markers of inflammation and acute phase were significantly reduced in the TPE group, and thus it was concluded that in the TPE group, patients had a faster clinical recovery [19]. This suggests that although all markers of inflammation are significantly reduced by TPE, the final results are not the desired ones. In the case of COVID-19 critically ill patients, the implementation of TPE under the mentioned circumstances could not restore the damaged pulmonary tissue and did not have a major impact on the improvement of other organ function. In patients with life-threatening COVID-19, TPE added to standard therapy compared with standard therapy alone resulted in clinical recovery but did not affect 35-day mortality, MSOF score, or the P/F ratio [19]. One of the limitations of our study is that although it includes a large number of patients, we did not use a control group, so we could not analyze the differences between the days of hospitalization and mortality.

Sultan Mehmood Kamran et al. [20] analyzed 45 patients who received TPE and 45 patients who did not receive TPE and found that the survival rate was higher in patients in whom TPE was initiated in the first 12 days after the onset of symptoms. They also observed that the duration of hospitalization was reduced in the group with TPE (10 days versus 15 days), and the mortality was higher (17.9%) in the group where TPE was performed later than 12 days after the onset of symptoms [20]. In our study, we observed that the average from the onset of symptoms until TPE was performed is 16.6 days. Thus, we can conclude that if TPE had been done earlier, the survival rate maybe would have been higher. This was difficult to achieve due to the epidemiological conditions and the large number of patients who needed admission in the hospital or in a place in ICU, in addition to late presentation to the hospital and to ICU.

Faryal Khamis et al. analyzed 31 patients with a mean age of 51 years, of whom 90% were men, 11 received TPE in the first two weeks of the disease, and 20 patients represented the control group [13]. They observed that in the TPE group mortality was significantly lower and the rate of extubating of patients was much higher (73% versus 20%), but the duration of hospitalization in intensive care was longer, with 14 days versus 6 days [13].

Cytokine storm is an aggressive inflammatory response acting through the release of an excessive amount of proinflammatory products [21]. It is correlated with interferon antagonism which inhibits the innate immune response, and it is directly proportional to lung injury, MSOF, and mortality [21].

In seven patients who had comorbidities such as hypertension (14.3%), asthma (14.3%), and diabetes (14.3%), Ikram Zaid et al. [22] obtained statistically significant results in the reduction in inflammatory markers and acute phase reactants (IL-6 p-value = 0.0004, fibrinogen p-value = 0.015, ferritin p-value = 0.011, and PCR p-value = 0.06), and all seven patients survived [22]. Our study clearly demonstrates a statistically significant decrease in biological markers (p-value: IL-6 < 0.0003, ferritin < 0.0001, fibrinogen < 0.0001, CRP = 0.0001, D-dimers = 0.0024, LDH < 0.001, and ESR < 0.0001), but the survival rate was much lower due to the large number of critical patients with more severe inflammatory markers and acute phase reactants compared with this study. The patients who received TPE in our hospital had a more critical situation. In our group, the average values for these markers before the first TPE session are even higher: IL-6 = 799 pg/mL, ferritin = 2364 μg/L, D-dimers = 5.18 μg/mL, CRP = 122 mg/L, LDH = 579 U/L, and fibrinogen = 4.90 g/L. We observed that using the TPE procedure in these cases can be a rescue procedure for the patients with severe ARDS forms (median P/F ratio 98.2).

Elimination of LDH is of particular importance, as its increase can be harmful by negatively impacting lactate levels, the activation of cytokines being an important marker of severity in the disease [23]. The same can be said for ferritin, IL-6 or CRP, as their increase plays a key role in inflammation [24].

Our study was conducted to evaluate the efficacy of TPE in patients with COVID-19 disease because critically ill patients had a high mortality rate due to the development of severe inflammatory syndrome and organ failure. Thus, Seyed Mohammad Reza Hashemian et al. [25] in a study of 15 patients (9 patients were male, and 6 patients were female), observed the efficacy of TPE by analyzing inflammatory cytokines, the PaO_2/FiO_2 ratio, and acute phase proteins. The ratio of biological markers in their study was significantly improved after the TPE session, where 9 (60%) of the 15 patients survived and 6 (40%) patients who needed mechanical ventilation died [25]. In our study of 65 patients

(45 were male, and 20 were female), we found that the survival rate was 24.6% (16 patients) and the rest of the patients who died developed multiple organ failure.

The plasma purification technique used in the studies published in the literature [13,20,26] was not different in terms of the volumes used or filters; the only thing that was used in various combinations was the substitution solution: albumin 5% and saline 0.9% [25], FFP [13,22], FFP and saline solution 0.9% [20], 5% albumin, and FFP [19], and no adverse reactions were observed to aggravate the clinical condition of the patients [13,19,20,22]. No adverse reactions were observed that aggravated the clinical condition of the patients [13,19,20,22]. No adverse reactions were observed in our study. We consider that TPE is a safe procedure in terms of side effects, and we have no reservations in initiating it from this point of view. On the other hand, in the worst case scenario, we can consider it a cosmetic maneuver to purify the patient's plasma, which is a breath of oxygen in the fight against COVID-19 disease. We consider that a favorable evolution in the critically ill patient with COVID-19 disease could be influenced even after the beginning of cytokine storm by associating other treatment options [26–28] such as antivirals, anti-inflammatory, immunomodulatory drugs, and anticoagulation [4,7,9], and by avoiding self-induced lung injury (SILI) by early intubation, followed by optimal protective mechanical ventilation [29,30]. The lung parenchyma compromised by inflammation and fibrosis cannot be restored by plasma clearance, but further damage might be stopped. TPE may be effective for reducing the systemic inflammation that could be involved in worsening the organ functions and may improve the outcome in patients with ARDS if it is started early [20].

A limitation of the study is that it is a retrospective uncontrolled single-center study, and we did not have a control group to analyze the difference between mortality and the number of days of hospitalization.

5. Conclusions

TPE can be used to reduce inflammation markers in COVID-19 critically ill patients and improve the PaO_2/FiO_2 ratio in patients with severe ARDS. This procedure also showed a minimum benefit in the survival of patients with extremely severe forms of COVID-19 disease. TPE should be used early with critically ill patients with ARDS. We consider that TPE and many other therapeutic approaches represent distinct pieces from the complicated puzzle of COVID-19 which still remains to be solved.

Author Contributions: Conceptualization, C.G. and T.M.P.; methodology, T.M.P. and C.G.; software, D.J.; validation, C.O., D.S. and I.O.S.; formal analysis, S.P., T.M.P. and C.G.; investigation, A.M. and A.-S.Z.; resources, S.P., V.L. and R.F.; data curation, D.J., S.P. and R.F.; writing—original draft preparation, C.G. and T.M.P.; writing—review and editing, C.L.Z.; visualization, L.A.N., A.-S.Z. and V.L.; supervision, C.O., I.O.S. and D.S.; project administration, T.M.P.; funding acquisition, C.G. All authors have read and agreed to the published version of the manuscript.

Funding: This research received no external funding.

Institutional Review Board Statement: The study was conducted in accordance with the Declaration of Helsinki and approved by the Ethics Committee of Emergency Clinical County Hospital (nr. 13037/24/12/2021).

Informed Consent Statement: Informed consent was obtained from all subjects involved in the study.

Data Availability Statement: Not applicable here.

Conflicts of Interest: The authors declare no conflict of interest.

References

1. Ranieri, V.M.; Rubenfeld, G.D.; Thompson, B.T.; Ferguson, N.D.; Caldwell, E.; Fan, E. Acute Respiratory Distress Syndrome: The Berlin Definition. *JAMA* **2012**, *307*, 2526–2533.
2. Seok Kim, J.; Young Lee, J.; Won Yang, J.; Hwa Lee, K.; Effenberger, M.; Szpirt, W. Immunopathogenesis and treatment of cytokine storm in COVID-19. *Theranostics* **2021**, *11*, 316–329.
3. Yavuz, S.; Ünal, S. Antiviral treatment of COVID-19. *Turk. J. Med. Sci.* **2020**, *50*, 611–619.

4. Ghasemnejad-Berenji, M.; Pashapour, S. Favipiravir and COVID-19: A Simplified Summary. *Drug Res.* **2021**, *71*, 166–170. [CrossRef] [PubMed]
5. Echeverría-Esnal, D.; Martin-Ontiyuelo, C.; Navarrete-Rouco, E.; De-Antonio Cuscó, M.; Ferrández, O. Azithromycin in the treatment of COVID-19: A review. *Expert. Rev. Anti-Infect Ther.* **2021**, *19*, 147–163. [CrossRef] [PubMed]
6. Khan, M.S.I.; Khan, M.S.I.; Debnath, C.R.; Nath, P.N.; Mahtab, M.; Nabeka, H. Ivermectin Treatment May Improve the Prognosis of Patients with COVID-19. *Arch. De Broncopneumol.* **2020**, *56*, 828–830.
7. Luo, P.; Liu, Y.; Qiu, L.; Liu, X.; Liu, D.; Li, J. Tocilizumab treatment in COVID-19: A single center experience. *J. Med. Virol.* **2020**, *92*, 814–818. [CrossRef]
8. Peter Horby, F.R.C.P.; Wei, S.L.; Jonathan, R.E.; Marion Mafham, M.D.; Jenifer Bell, L. Dexamethasone in Hospitalized Patients with COVID-19. *N. Engl. J. Med.* **2021**, *384*, 693–704. [PubMed]
9. Hadid, T.; Kafri, Z.; Al-Katib, A. Coagulation and anticoagulation in COVID-19. *Blood Rev.* **2021**, *47*, 100–112. [CrossRef]
10. Tabibi, S.; Tabibi, T.Z.; Conic, R.R.; Banisaeed, N.; Streiff, M.B. Therapeutic Plasma Exchange: A potential Management Strategy for Critically Ill COVID-19 Patients. *J. Intensive Care Med.* **2020**, *35*, 827–835. [CrossRef]
11. Lu, W.; Kelley, W.; Fang, D.C.; Joshi, S.; Kim, Y.; Paroder, M. The use of therapeutic plasma exchange as adjunctive therapy in the treatment of coronavirus disease 2019: A critical appraisal of the current evidence. *J. Clin. Apher.* **2021**, *36*, 483–491. [CrossRef] [PubMed]
12. Lyu, R.K.; Chen, W.H.; Hsieh, S.T. Plasma Exchange Versus Double Filtration Plasmapheresis in the Treatment of Guillain-Barré Syndrome. *Ther. Apher.* **2002**, *6*, 163–166. [CrossRef]
13. Khamis, F.; Al-Zakwani, I.; Al Hashmi, S.; Al Dowaiki, S.; Al Bahrani, M.; Pandak, N. Therapeutic plasma exchange in adults with severe COVID-19 infection. *Int. J. Infect. Dis.* **2020**, *99*, 214–218. [CrossRef]
14. Moore, J.B.; June, C.H. Cytokine release syndrome in severe COVID-19. *Science* **2020**, *368*, 473–474. [CrossRef] [PubMed]
15. Blot, M.; Bour, J.B.; Quenot, J.P.; Bourredjem, A.; Nguyen, M.; Guy, J. The dysregulated innate immune response in severe COVID-19 pneumonia that could drive poorer outcome. *J. Transl. Med.* **2020**, *18*, 457. [CrossRef] [PubMed]
16. Zhang, L.; Zhai, H.; Ma, S.; Chen, J.; Gao, Y. Efficacy of therapeutic plasma exchange in severe COVID-19 patients. *Br. J. Haematol.* **2020**, *190*, 181–183. [CrossRef]
17. Biban, P.; Standage, S.W.; Jayashree, M.; Samprathi, M. Biomarkers in COVID-19: An Up-To-Date Review. *Rev. Front. Pediatr.* **2020**, *8*, 607–647.
18. Krzych, Ł.J.; Putowski, Z.; Czok, M.; Hofman, M.; Fraaij, P.L. What Is the Role of Therapeutic Plasma Exchange as an Adjunctive Treatment in Severe COVID-19: A Systematic Review. *Viruses* **2021**, *13*, 1484. [CrossRef]
19. Faqihi, F.; Alharthy, A.; Abdulaziz, S.; Balhamar, A.; Alomari, A.; Al Aseri, Z. Therapeutic plasma exchange in patients with life-threatening COVID-19: A randomised controlled clinical trial. *Int. J. Antimicrob. Agents* **2021**, *57*, 106334. [CrossRef]
20. Kamran, M.; Mirza, Z.E.H.; Naseem, A.; Liaqat, J.; Fazal, I.; Alamgir, W. Therapeutic plasma exchange for coronavirus disease-2019 triggered cytokine release syndrome: A retrospective propensity matched control study. *PLoS ONE* **2021**, *16*, 0244853. [CrossRef]
21. Behrens, E.M.; Koretzky, G.A. Cytokine Storm Syndrome Looking Toward the Precision Medicine Era. *Arthritis Rheumatol.* **2017**, *69*, 1135–1143. [CrossRef]
22. Zaid, I.; Essaad, O.; El Aidouni, G.; Aabdi, M.; Berrichi, S.; Taouihar, S. Therapeutic plasma exchange in patients with COVID-19 pneumonia in intensive care unit: Cases series. *Ann. Med. Surg.* **2021**, *71*, 102920. [CrossRef] [PubMed]
23. Lionte, C.; Sorodoc, V.; Haliga, R.E.; Bologa, C.; Ceasovschih, A.; Petris, O.R.; Coman, A.E.; Stoica, A.; Sirbu, O.; Puha, G.; et al. Inflammatory and Cardiac Biomarkers in Relation with Post-Acute COVID-19 and Mortality: What We Know after Succesive Pandemic Vawes. *Diagnostics* **2022**, *12*, 1373. [CrossRef]
24. Brandon Michael Henry, M.; Gaurav, A.; Johnny, W. Lactate dehydrogenase levels predict coronavirus disease 2019 (COVID-19) severity and mortality: A pooled analysis. *Am. J. Emerg. Med.* **2020**, *38*, 1722–1726. [CrossRef] [PubMed]
25. Hashemian, S.M.; Shafigh, N.; Afzal, G.; Jamaati, H.; Tabarsi, P.; Marjani, M. Plasmapheresis reduces cytokine and immune cell levels in COVID-19 patients with acute respiratory distress syndrome (ARDS). *Pulmonology* **2021**, *27*, 486–492. [CrossRef] [PubMed]
26. Furong, Z.; Yuzhao, H.; Ying, G.; Mingzhu, Y. Association of inflammatory markers with the severity of COVID-19: A meta-analysis. *Int. J. Infect. Dis.* **2020**, *96*, 467–474.
27. Haliga, R.E.; Sorodoc, V.; Lionte, C.; Petris, O.; Bologa, C.; Coman, A.E.; Vata, L.G.; Puha, G.; Dumitrescu, G.; Sirbu, O.; et al. Acute clinical Syndromes and Suspicion of SARS-CoV-2 Infection. The Experience of a Single Romanian Center in the early Pandemic Period. *Medicina* **2021**, *57*, 121. [CrossRef]
28. Truong, A.D.; Auld, S.C.; Barker, N.A.; Friend, S.; Wynn, A.; Thanushi Cobb, J. Therapeutic plasma exchange for COVID-19-associated hyperviscosity. *Transfusion* **2021**, *61*, 1029–1034. [CrossRef]
29. Gavriatopoulou, M.; Ntanasis-Stathopoulos, I.; Korompoki, E.; Fotiou, D.; Migkou, M.; Tzannnis, I.G. Emerging treatment strategies for COVID-19 infection. *Clin. Exp. Med.* **2021**, *21*, 167–179. [CrossRef]
30. Gosangi, B.; Rubinowitz, A.N.; David, I.; Gange, C.; Bader, A.; Cortopassi, I. COVID-19 ARDS: A review of imaging features and overview of mechanical ventilation and its complications. *Emerg. Radiol.* **2022**, *29*, 23–34. [CrossRef]

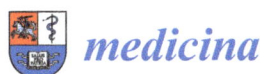

Case Report

A Case of a Malignant Lymphoma Patient Persistently Infected with SARS-CoV-2 for More than 6 Months

Yoji Nagasaki [1,*], Masanori Kadowaki [2], Asako Nakamura [3], Yoshiki Etoh [3], Masatoshi Shimo [2], Sayoko Ishihara [1], Yoko Arimizu [1], Rena Iwamoto [4], Seiji Kamamuta [4] and Hiromi Iwasaki [2]

[1] Department of Infectious Disease, Clinical Research Institute, National Hospital Organization Kyushu Medical Center, Fukuoka 8108563, Japan
[2] Department of Hematology, Clinical Research Institute, National Hospital Organization Kyushu Medical Center, Fukuoka 8108563, Japan
[3] Fukuoka Institute of Health and Environmental Sciences, Fukuoka 8180135, Japan
[4] Department of Clinical Laboratory, Clinical Research Institute, National Hospital Organization Kyushu Medical Center, Fukuoka 8108563, Japan
* Correspondence: nagasaki.yoji.up@mail.hosp.go.jp; Tel.:+81-92-852-0700

Abstract: Coronavirus disease 2019 (COVID-19) is an emerging infectious disease caused by severe acute respiratory syndrome 2 (SARS-CoV-2). There are many unknowns regarding the handling of long-term SARS-CoV-2 infections in immunocompromised patients. Here, we describe the lethal disease course in a SARS-CoV-2-infected patient during Bruton's tyrosine kinase inhibitor therapy. We performed whole-genome analysis using samples obtained during the course of the disease in a 63-year-old woman who was diagnosed with intraocular malignant lymphoma of the right eye in 2012. She had received treatment since the diagnosis. An autologous transplant was performed in 2020, but she experienced a worsening of the primary disease 26 days before she was diagnosed with a positive SARS-CoV-2 RT-PCR. Tirabrutinib was administered for the primary disease. A cluster of COVID-19 infections occurred in the hematological ward while the patient was hospitalized, and she became infected on day 0. During the course of the disease, she experienced repeated remission exacerbations of COVID-19 pneumonia and eventually died on day 204. SARS-CoV-2 whole-viral sequencing revealed that the patient shed the virus long-term. Viral infectivity studies confirmed infectious virus on day 189, suggesting that the patient might be still infectious. This case report describes the duration and viral genetic evaluation of a patient with malignant lymphoma who developed SARS-CoV-2 infection during Bruton's tyrosine kinase inhibitor therapy and in whom the infection persisted for over 6 months.

Keywords: SARS-CoV-2; immunocompromised host; Bruton's tyrosine kinase; persistent infection

Citation: Nagasaki, Y.; Kadowaki, M.; Nakamura, A.; Etoh, Y.; Shimo, M.; Ishihara, S.; Arimizu, Y.; Iwamoto, R.; Kamamuta, S.; Iwasaki, H. A Case of a Malignant Lymphoma Patient Persistently Infected with SARS-CoV-2 for More than 6 Months. *Medicina* 2023, 59, 108. https://doi.org/10.3390/medicina59010108

Academic Editor: Patrick Geraghty

Received: 9 December 2022
Revised: 25 December 2022
Accepted: 28 December 2022
Published: 4 January 2023

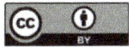

Copyright: © 2023 by the authors. Licensee MDPI, Basel, Switzerland. This article is an open access article distributed under the terms and conditions of the Creative Commons Attribution (CC BY) license (https://creativecommons.org/licenses/by/4.0/).

1. Introduction

Despite the introduction of coronavirus disease 2019 (COVID-19) mRNA vaccines, severe acute respiratory syndrome coronavirus 2 (SARS-CoV-2) continues to mutate and remains as major threat to immunocompromised hosts. Immunocompromised people have an increased risk of developing severe COVID-19 outcomes [1] and might not acquire the same level of protection from COVID-19 vaccines compared with immunocompetent hosts [2]. The adverse outcomes associated with COVID-19 infection in patients with hematological malignancies stem at least in part from intrinsic immune dysfunction [3]. Hematological patients experience delayed viral clearance, which results in persistent shedding of viable SARS-CoV-2 and the emergence of multiple mutations [4].

Whether and for how long immunocompromised patients shed infectious virus has profound implications for understanding disease transmission and treatment for hematological patents. A recent case report showed prolonged infectious SARS-CoV-2 shedding for 143 days post-symptom onset in an immunocompromised patient [5]. However, the detection of viral genomic material does not confirm the presence of infectious SARS-CoV-2.

The duration of infectiousness and, consequently, the necessary duration of isolation in healthcare institutions, are unanswered questions. The United States Centers for Diseases Control and Prevention recommends a 5 day isolation period for COVID-19 patients with mild illness who have been fever free for at least 24 h. This period is extended to up to 10 days for patients with severe infection and/or severe immunosuppression. Ending isolation without a viral test may not be an option in these cases [6].

Here, we describe the lethal disease course in a persistently SARS-CoV-2-infected patient for more than 6 months during Bruton's tyrosine kinase (BTK) inhibitor therapy. We performed whole-genome analysis using samples obtained during the course of the patient's disease.

2. Materials and Methods

2.1. Saliva and Nasopharyngeal Reverse Transcription Polymerase Chain Reaction (RT-PCR) Testing

Salivary or nasopharyngeal samples were collected from the patient, as follows: T1 (Day 0), T2 (Day 34), T3 (Day 43), T4 (Day 49), T5 (Day 55), T6 (Day 78), T7 (Day 107), T8 (Day 114), T9 (Day 128), T10 (Day 135), T11 (Day 140), and T12 (Day 189). The samples underwent RT-PCR testing for SARS-CoV-2 with the Ampdirect™ 2019-nCoV detection kit (Shimadzu Corporation, Kyoto, Japan), in which two sequences specific to SARS-CoV-2, N1 and N2, as defined by the United States Centers for Disease Control and Prevention, were targeted as primers and probes [7]. The real-time PCR analyzer for the SARS-CoV-2 diagnosis was the cobas® z 480 (Roche Diagnostics, Basel Switzerland) or the QIAamp Viral RNA Mini QIAcube Kit (Qiqgen GMBH, Hilden, Germany) which showed that N1 and N2 were amplified, with cycle threshold values of approximately 40. All samples were frozen at $-80\ °C$ after the SARS-CoV-2 RT-PCR test was performed.

2.2. Serological Testing for SARS-CoV-2 Antibody

Serological testing for antibodies targeting the S1 subunit of the viral spike protein (Immunoglobulin G, spike protein receptor-binding domain) and antibodies targeting the viral nucleocapsid protein (Immunoglobulin G, nucleocapsid protein) was performed at Roche using the Elecsys® Anti-SARS-CoV-2 S test and Elecsys® Anti-SARS-CoV-2 test (Roche Diagnostics), respectively.

2.3. SARS-CoV-2 Whole Viral Sequencing and Phylogenetic Analysis

The nucleotide sequences of SARS-CoV-2 obtained from nasopharyngeal swabs or saliva collected from the patient were evaluated at nine time points, as follows: T1 (Day 0), T2 (Day 34), T3 (Day 43), T4 (Day 49), T5 (Day 55), T9 (Day 128), T10 (Day 135), T11 (Day 140), and T12 (Day 189). The whole-genome sequencing of SARS-CoV-2 was performed using the method of Itokawa et al. [8] based on the ARTIC Network's multiplex PCR (https://artic.network/ncov-2019, accessed on 6 April 2021). The resulting DNA libraries were sequenced with the MiSeq system (Illumina, San Diego, CA, USA).

Sequence reads were analyzed by the method of Sekizuka et al. [9] to obtain the whole genome sequence. The patient's viral sequences can be located with Global Initiative on Sharing All Influenza Data (GISAID) [10], accession numbers EPI_ISL_15610661, EPI_ISL_15610675, EPI_ISL_15610808, EPI_ISL_15610828, EPI_ISL_15610943, EPI_ISL_15610944, EPI_ISL_15610971, EPI_ISL_15610972, and EPI_ISL_2015094.

The comparison dataset comprised 27 representative SARS-CoV-2 genomes selected from Nextstrain (https://nextstrain.org/, accessed on 17 August 2022) by regions of interest (Japan, Asia, Europe, North and South America). Furthermore, 30 sequences representative of Fukuoka Prefecture, Japan, were selected from the GISAID database.

These reference sequences and those obtained from the patient, in addition to Wuhan-Hu-1, NC_045512.2 were aligned using multiple alignment using fast Fourier transform (MAFFT) software ver.7 (https://mafft.cbrc.jp/alignment/software/tips.html, accessed on 23 August 2022). The best-fit substitution model for the maximum likelihood method was selected using MEGA.11 software (https://www.megasoftware.net/, accessed on 23 August 2022). Maximum likelihood phylogenetic trees were created using the general time reversible plus G substitution (GTR+G) model with 1000 bootstrap replicates (Tables S1 and S2).

2.4. SARS-CoV-2 Viral Infectivity Studies

Specimens were centrifuged at 3000 rpm for 15 min. The supernatant was filtered through a 0.22 μm filter (Millipore; Sigma-Aldrich, Madrid, Spain) then diluted 1:3 in Dulbecco's modified Eagle's medium (D-MEM) (Wako, Osaka, Japan). Next, 50 μL of the diluted sample was added to Vero-E6/TMPRESS cells (Japanese Collection of Research Bioresources Cell Bank; https://cellbank.nibiohn.go.jp/english/, accessed on 23 August 2022) in a 12 well plate. The plate was then incubated for 1 h at 37 °C in a 5% carbon dioxide incubator. After 1 h, the inoculum was removed and washed twice with D-MEM, and then D-MEM with 2% of fetal bovine serum was added at 37 °C in a 5% carbon dioxide incubator. Cells were then incubated for an additional 9 days.

3. Case

The patient, a 63-year-old female, was diagnosed with intraocular malignant lymphoma of the right eye in 2012 and began treatment. The lesion later spread to the central nervous system (CNS), and she was treated continuously throughout repeated hospital admissions and discharges. An autologous transplant was performed in 2020 to control the disease. She was later admitted to the hematology ward for rescue therapy owing to a worsening of the primary disease 26 days before she was diagnosed with a positive SARS-CoV-2 RT-PCR. Tirabrutinib was administered for the primary disease on the same day, with a partial response. A cluster of COVID-19 infections occurred in the hematological ward while the patient was hospitalized. At this point, her SARS-CoV-2 RT-PCR test result was negative; however, a fever and sore throat developed 4 days later, and the test result was positive on day 0. We define her initial day of presentation with SARS-CoV-2 RT-PCR positive as day 0 of COIVD-19 infection. Because the designated ward for COVID-19 patients in our hospital had reached its full capacity, the patient was transferred to another hospital for treatment from day 1. Chest computed tomography (CT) was performed at the time of transfer, which showed ground glass opacities (GGO) in the upper lobe of the left lung. Tirabrutinib was discontinued from day 3, and the patient was treated with remdesivir for 5 days. She was transferred back to our hospital on day 17 for continued treatment for the malignant lymphoma, as her condition was good despite continued temperatures of 37.2–37.8 °C. Soon after her return, she gradually developed a temperature above 38 °C and hypoxemia. Methylprednisolone (mPSL, 1 mg/kg) was administered on day 28 owing to an immune response after the COVID-19 infection. Chest CT findings on day 30 showed extensive GGO with contractile changes and infiltrative shadows, and the hypoxemia had worsened. On day 32, tocilizumab and mPSL (500 mg) were administered for their anti-inflammatory effects. However, the pneumonia worsened on day 34. Additionally, the SARS-CoV-2 RT-PCR test results had remained positive since the diagnosis. A second course of remdesivir was administered for 5 days from day 34 onwards, considering a relapse of COVID-19. Thereafter, her condition gradually improved, and the steroid dosage was tapered by 10 mg each week. Tirabrutinib was resumed to control the malignant lymphoma. However, on day 70, head magnetic resonance imaging revealed worsening of the CNS lesions of malignant lymphoma, and whole-brain irradiation was initiated for life-saving purposes. The patient's consciousness gradually improved, and she was able to eat. However, the suspected complication of aspiration pneumonia was discovered; therefore, antimicrobial agents were administered. On day 110, chest CT again showed pneumonia with GGO in both lungs. Interstitial pneumonia due to COVID-19 or drug-induced pneumonia was considered. On the same day, mPSL (250 mg) was re-administered. As the pneumonia improved, prednisolone (1 mg/kg) was maintained thereafter. However, leukoencephalopathy was identified after radiotherapy, and the patient was discharged and returned home on day 147 to receive palliative care. During the patient's hospitalization, she never tested negative for SARS-CoV-2 with RT-PCR, and she was negative for antibody production (Figure 1). During home care, hypoxemia progressed on day 189. SARS-CoV-2 RT-PCR was performed, and the result was positive. The patient died on day 204 (Figures 1 and 2).

SARS-CoV-2 RT-PCR-positive samples were used to analyze the genetic mutations during the course of the patient's disease. Twelve samples (T1–12) were analyzed; T6, T7, and T8 samples could not be analyzed owing to low viral load. Whole-genome sequences were examined for mutational transitions compared with the T1 sequences. As a result: T2 sample, three mutations; T3 sample, five mutations; T4 and T5 samples, one mutation; T9, T10, and T11 samples, five mutations; T12 sample, seven mutations (Figure 3). Over time, whole viral sequencing revealed the development of seven mutations. Viral infectivity studies were performed using all 12 samples. Only the T12 sample confirmed the presence of infectious virus.

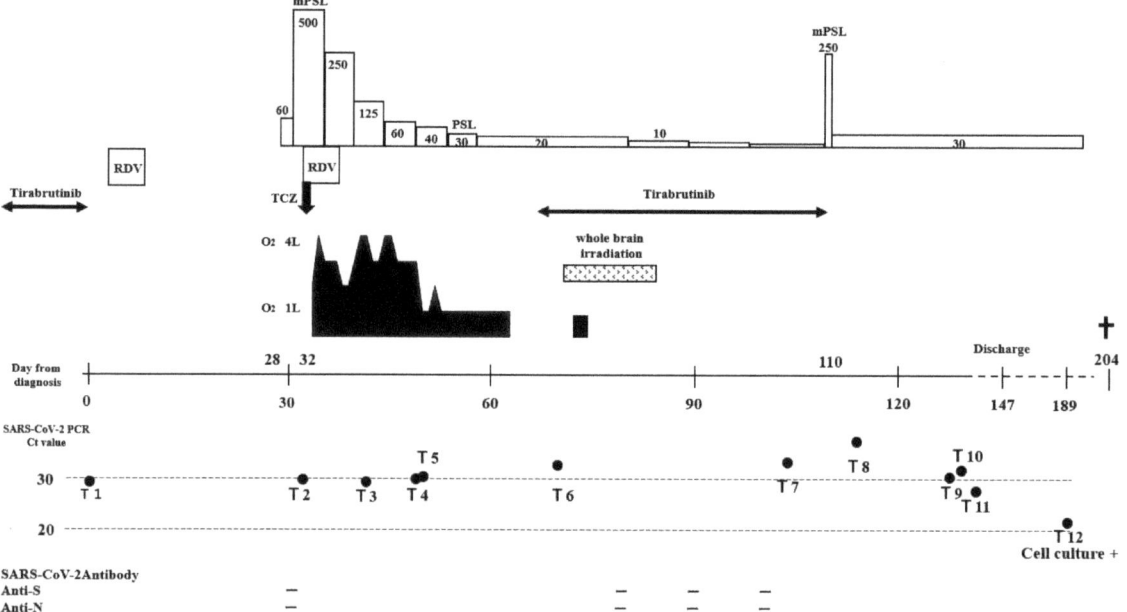

Figure 1. The clinical course of the patient and the time course of the levels of SARS-CoV-2 viral RNA and the results of antibody testing. SARS-CoV-2: severe acute respiratory syndrome coronavirus 2; RDV: remdesivir; TCZ: tocilizumab; mPSL: methylprednisolone; PSL: prednisolone; Ct: cycle threshold, Anti-S; antibody spike protein; Anti-N, antibody nucleocapsid protein.

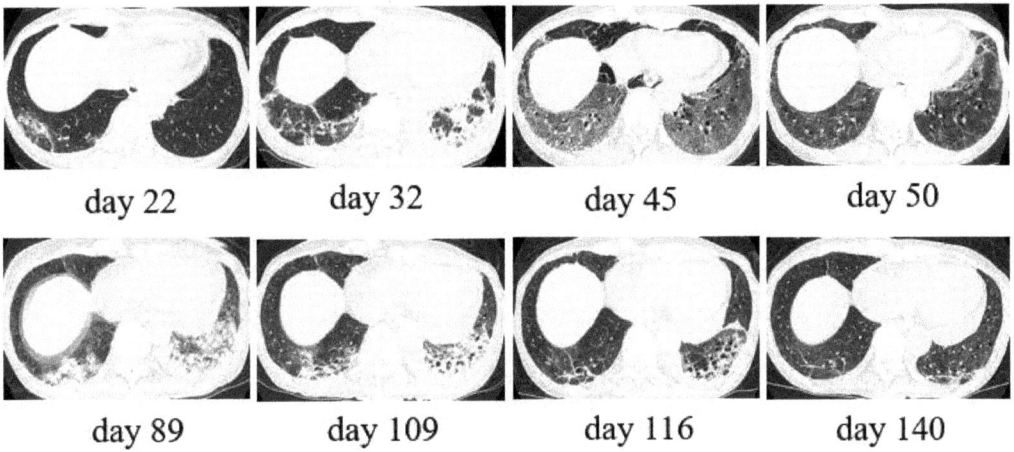

Figure 2. Representative chest computed tomography (CT) image at the level of the lower lobe bronchus.

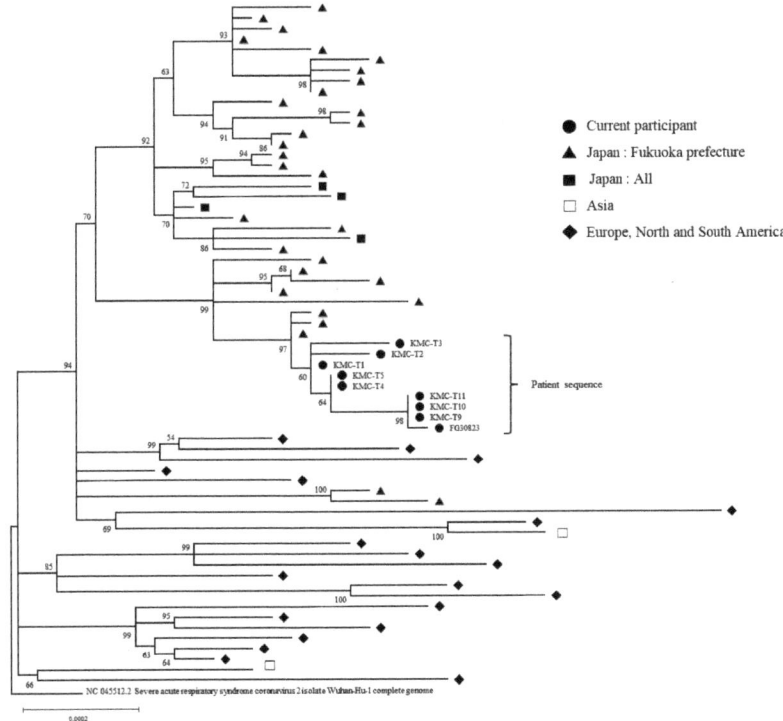

Figure 3. Phylogenetic analysis of SARS-CoV-2 whole-genome virus nucleotide sequences from longitudinally collected nasopharyngeal swab or saliva specimens. Phylogenetic trees were constructed by the maximum likelihood method. Nucleotide sequences of SARS-CoV-2 were obtained from nasopharyngeal swabs or saliva that were collected from the patient at nine time points (●; T1, T2, T3, T4, T5, T9, T10, T11, and T12). Sequences were collected from samples from Fukuoka Prefecture, Japan (▲) and all regions in Japan (■), Asia and Europe (□), and North and South America (◆), as reference sequences. The scale represents 0.0002 nucleotide substitutions per site.

4. Discussion

The patient described in this case report, with intraocular malignant lymphoma and CNS recurrence, contracted COVID-19 while taking tirabrutinib. Thereafter, shedding of viable SARS-CoV-2 persisted for approximately 6 months, with repeated episodes of COVID-19 pneumonia. The result of the SARS-CoV-2 RT-PCR tests performed during the course of the patient's hospitalization were never negative, and there was no SARS-CoV-2 antibody production. Whole-viral sequencing analysis of the samples during the study suggested that the same virus persisted, with repeated mutations and persistent infectiousness.

There are many reports of immunocompromised persons shedding SARS-CoV-2 for long periods of time [4,5,11–14]. One of these reported cases is that of Choi et al. [5] who detected SARS-CoV-2 up to 143 days after infection. The reason for the persistent infection was thought to be the repeated administration of immunosuppressive drugs to control severe antiphospholipid antibody syndrome with alveolar hemorrhage. Factors associated with delayed SARS-CoV-2 clearance include, but are not limited to, older age, severe disease, multiple underlying diseases, immunocompromised status, hematological diseases that involve transplantation, and transplantation for solid tumors [15,16]. The following factors were considered to have contributed to the persistent infection in this case: (1) latent immunodeficiency after auto-transplantation, (2) immunosuppressive state induced by oral tirabrutinib, and (3) repeated administration of steroids.

COVID-19 is a biphasic illness with an initial viremic phase and a later effective adaptive immune phase [17]. Therefore, treatment of COVID-19 depends on the phase. It makes sense to administer neutralizing antibody products and antiviral drugs during the viremic phase and anti-inflammatory drugs during the later effective adaptive immune phase. The timing of anti-inflammatory drug administration is especially important because severe COVID-19 is caused by cytokine storms [17]. Some studies describe disadvantages of immunosuppressive therapy and indicate a delay in viral clearance in immunosuppressed conditions [18,19]. Hematological malignancies are biologically heterogeneous with a spectrum of inherent immune impairment that is further exacerbated by disease-directed therapies. Additionally, antibody production capacity is reduced, which makes it difficult to eliminate the virus, resulting in higher mortality rates [3,20].

Our patient was treated with tirabrutinib for refractory primary CNS lymphoma. Ibrutinib was promptly discontinued owing to concerns about B-cell dysfunction when COVID-19 infection was confirmed. Ibrutinib is a potent, covalent inhibitor of BTK, a kinase downstream of the B-cell receptor that is critical for B-cell survival and proliferation [21,22]. BTK inhibitors, which target a wide range of proinflammatory signaling pathways, may play a key role in the management of COVID-19 [23]. However, it has been suggested that these drugs may be unsuitable for viral elimination because they suppress antibody production by inhibiting B-cell function [24]. Another report describes the ability of Burton kinase inhibitor-treated patients to produce antibodies after vaccination against SARS-CoV-2. The response rate for these patients who received active Burton kinase inhibitors was very low (23%) [25]. In our case, the administration of a BTK inhibitor and steroids suppressed the excessive immune response. However, it is possible that the patient was unable to eliminate the virus owing to a failure to produce antibodies against SARS-CoV-2. As a result, although the patient did not develop severe pneumonia, SARS-CoV-2 was not eliminated, and she was considered to be persistently infectious, with the virus continuing to mutate.

Phylogenetic analysis results over 6 months in this case had a common ancestor. The different sequences and phylogeny of the same area detected at the same time suggested persistent infection rather than reinfection. As mentioned above, it was proven that the decreased ability to produce antibodies following treatment with BTK inhibitor and steroids made it difficult for our patient to eliminate SARS-CoV-2, resulting in repeated replication, which led to persistent infection. Furthermore, the fact that cells could be isolated from the specimens prior to death means that infectivity was sustained.

As in this report, uncertainty continues regarding COVID-19 de-isolation of immunocompromised hosts. Patients should be considered infectious and quarantined during the period of viral shedding. Usually, cell culture methods are not used to determine the end of isolation. Viral culture positivity may also not correlate perfectly with transmissibility, although the correlation between culture data and PCR cycle threshold values may help predict infectiousness [26]. Further data are needed to understand the correlation between transmission risk, culture positivity, and PCR cycle threshold values. However, there are various problems with the stability of the test, such as sampling errors. The presence or absence of symptoms is also important, but there is essentially no other way to address the issue of de-isolation than comply with infection control measures. Above all, it is important to vaccinate and administer antibody products to immunocompromised persons as a means of preventing infection [3].

5. Conclusions

This case report describes the duration and genetic study of a patient with malignant lymphoma who was infected with SARS-CoV-2 during BTK inhibitor therapy and who sustained persistent infection for over 6 months. This report provides evidence that B-cell function might play a key role in resolving COVID-19 infection.

Supplementary Materials: The following are available online at www.mdpi.com/xxx/S1, Table S1: Worldwide representative SARS-CoV-2 sequences registered in GISAID (https://www.gisaid.org) from September 2020 to March 2021, Table S2: Representative SARS-CoV-2 sequence from Fukuoka Prefecture, Japan registered in GISAID (https://www.gisaid.org) from September 2020 to March 2021.

Author Contributions: Conceptualization, Y.N.; data curation, Y.N., M.K., R.I., S.K., M.S., S.I., Y.A., and A.N.; writing—original draft preparation, Y.N.; writing—review and editing, Y.N., A.N., and Y.E. with support from H.I. All authors have read and agreed to the published version of the manuscript.

Funding: This report received no external funding.

Institutional Review Board Statement: This study was approved by the Institutional Review Board of the National Hospital Organization Kyushu Medical Center (approval number 20C164; 25 November 2020).

Informed Consent Statement: Informed consent was obtained from all subjects involved in the study. Written informed consent has been obtained from the patient to publish this paper.

Data Availability Statement: The data presented in this study are available on request from the corresponding author.

Conflicts of Interest: The authors declare no conflict of interest.

References

1. Williamson, E.J.; Walker, A.J.; Bhaskaran, K.; Bacon, S.; Bates, C.; Morton, C.E.; Curtis, H.J.; Mehrkar, A.; Evans, D.; Inglesby, P.; et al. Factors associated with COVID-19-related death using OpenSAFELY. *Nature* **2020**, *584*, 430–436. [CrossRef] [PubMed]
2. Tenforde, M.W.; Patel, M.M.; Ginde, A.A.; Douin, D.J.; Talbot, H.K.; Casey, J.D.; Mohr, N.M.; Zepeski, A.; Gaglani, M.; McNeal, T.; et al. Effectiveness of Severe Acute Respiratory Syndrome Coronavirus 2 Messenger RNA Vaccines for Preventing Coronavirus Disease 2019 Hospitalizations in the United States. *Clin. Infect. Dis.* **2022**, *74*, 1515–1524. [CrossRef] [PubMed]
3. Langerbeins, P.; Hallek, M. COVID-19 in patients with hematologic malignancy. *Blood* **2022**, *140*, 236–252. [CrossRef] [PubMed]
4. Leung, W.F.; Chorlton, S.; Tyson, J.; Al-Rawahi, G.N.; Jassem, A.N.; Prystajecky, N.; Masud, S.; Deans, G.D.; Chapman, M.G. COVID-19 in an immunocompromised host: Persistent shedding of viable SARS-CoV-2 and emergence of multiple mutations: A case report. *Int. J. Infect. Dis.* **2022**, *114*, 178–182. [CrossRef]
5. Choi, B.; Choudhary, M.C.; Regan, J.; Sparks, J.A.; Padera, R.F.; Qiu, X.; Solomon, I.H.; Kuo, H.H.; Boucau, J.; Bowman, K.; et al. Persistence and Evolution of SARS-CoV-2 in an Immunocompromised Host. *N. Engl. J. Med.* **2020**, *383*, 2291–2293. [CrossRef]
6. Prevenstion CfDCa. *Isolation and Precaution for People with COVID-19*; CDC: Atlanta, GA, USA, 2022.
7. Lee, J.S.; Goldstein, J.M.; Moon, J.L.; Herzegh, O.; Bagarozzi, D.A., Jr.; Oberste, M.S.; Hughes, H.; Bedi, K.; Gerard, D.; Cameron, B.; et al. Analysis of the initial lot of the CDC 2019-Novel Coronavirus (2019-nCoV) real-time RT-PCR diagnostic panel. *PLoS ONE* **2021**, *16*, e0260487. [CrossRef]
8. Itokawa, K.; Sekizuka, T.; Hashino, M.; Tanaka, R.; Kuroda, M. Disentangling primer interactions improves SARS-CoV-2 genome sequencing by multiplex tiling PCR. *PLoS ONE* **2020**, *15*, e0239403. [CrossRef]

9. Sekizuka, T.; Itokawa, K.; Hashino, M.; Kawano-Sugaya, T.; Tanaka, R.; Yatsu, K.; Ohnishi, A.; Goto, K.; Tsukagoshi, H.; Ehara, H.; et al. A Genome Epidemiological Study of SARS-CoV-2 Introduction into Japan. *mSphere* **2020**, *5*, e00786-20. [CrossRef]
10. Shu, Y.; McCauley, J. GISAID: Global initiative on sharing all influenza data—From vision to reality. *Eurosurveillance* **2017**, *22*, 30494. [CrossRef]
11. Tarhini, H.; Recoing, A.; Bridier-Nahmias, A.; Rahi, M.; Lambert, C.; Martres, P.; Lucet, J.C.; Rioux, C.; Bouzid, D.; Lebourgeois, S.; et al. Long-Term Severe Acute Respiratory Syndrome Coronavirus 2 (SARS-CoV-2) Infectiousness Among Three Immunocompromised Patients: From Prolonged Viral Shedding to SARS-CoV-2 Superinfection. *J. Infect. Dis.* **2021**, *223*, 1522–1527. [CrossRef]
12. Avanzato, V.A.; Matson, M.J.; Seifert, S.N.; Pryce, R.; Williamson, B.N.; Anzick, S.L.; Barbian, K.; Judson, S.D.; Fischer, E.R.; Martens, C.; et al. Case Study: Prolonged Infectious SARS-CoV-2 Shedding from an Asymptomatic Immunocompromised Individual with Cancer. *Cell* **2020**, *183*, 1901–1912.e9. [CrossRef]
13. Camprubí, D.; Gaya, A.; Marcos, M.A.; Martí-Soler, H.; Soriano, A.; del Mar Mosquera, M.; Oliver, A.; Santos, M.; Muñoz, J.; García-Vidal, C. Persistent replication of SARS-CoV-2 in a severely immunocompromised patient treated with several courses of remdesivir. *Int. J. Infect. Dis.* **2021**, *104*, 379–381. [CrossRef] [PubMed]
14. Sepulcri, C.; Dentone, C.; Mikulska, M.; Bruzzone, B.; Lai, A.; Fenoglio, D.; Bozzano, F.; Bergna, A.; Parodi, A.; Altosole, T.; et al. The Longest Persistence of Viable SARS-CoV-2 With Recurrence of Viremia and Relapsing Symptomatic COVID-19 in an Immunocompromised Patient-A Case Study. *Open Forum Infect Dis.* **2021**, *8*, ofab217. [CrossRef] [PubMed]
15. Aydillo, T.; Gonzalez-Reiche, A.S.; Aslam, S.; van de Guchte, A.; Khan, Z.; Obla, A.; Dutta, J.; van Bakel, H.; Aberg, J.; García-Sastre, A.; et al. Shedding of Viable SARS-CoV-2 after Immunosuppressive Therapy for Cancer. *N. Engl. J. Med.* **2020**, *383*, 2586–2588. [CrossRef] [PubMed]
16. Epstein, R.L.; Sperring, H.; Hofman, M.; Lodi, S.; White, L.F.; Barocas, J.A.; Bouton, T.C.; Xiao, Y.; Hsu, H.E.; Miller, N.S.; et al. Time to SARS-CoV-2 PCR Clearance in Immunocompromising Conditions: Is Test-Based Removal From Isolation Necessary in Severely Immunocompromised Individuals? *Open Forum. Infect. Dis.* **2021**, *8*, ofab164. [CrossRef]
17. García, L.F. Immune Response, Inflammation, and the Clinical Spectrum of COVID-19. *Front. Immunol.* **2020**, *11*, 1441. [CrossRef]
18. Arora, K.; Panda, P.K. Steroid harms if given early in COVID-19 viraemia. *BMJ Case Rep.* **2021**, *14*, e241105. [CrossRef]
19. Fishman, J.A.; Grossi, P.A. Novel Coronavirus-19 (COVID-19) in the immunocompromised transplant recipient: #Flatteningthecurve. *Am. J. Transplant.* **2020**, *20*, 1765–1767.
20. Passamonti, F.; Cattaneo, C.; Arcaini, L.; Bruna, R.; Cavo, M.; Merli, F.; Angelucci, E.; Krampera, M.; Cairoli, R.; Della Porta, M.G.; et al. Clinical characteristics and risk factors associated with COVID-19 severity in patients with haematological malignancies in Italy: A retrospective, multicentre, cohort study. *Lancet Haematol.* **2020**, *7*, e737–e745. [CrossRef]
21. Jacobs, C.F.; Eldering, E.; Kater, A.P. Kinase inhibitors developed for treatment of hematologic malignancies: Implications for immune modulation in COVID-19. *Blood Adv.* **2021**, *5*, 913–925. [CrossRef]
22. Davids, M.S.; Brown, J.R. Ibrutinib: A first in class covalent inhibitor of Bruton's tyrosine kinase. *Future Oncol.* **2014**, *10*, 957–967. [CrossRef] [PubMed]
23. Kifle, Z.D. Bruton tyrosine kinase inhibitors as potential therapeutic agents for COVID-19: A review. *Metab. Open* **2021**, *11*, 100116. [CrossRef] [PubMed]
24. Chung, D.J.; Shah, G.L.; Devlin, S.M.; Ramanathan, L.V.; Doddi, S.; Pessin, M.S.; Hoover, E.; Marcello, L.T.; Young, J.C.; Boutemine, S.R.; et al. Disease- and Therapy-Specific Impact on Humoral Immune Responses to COVID-19 Vaccination in Hematologic Malignancies. *Blood Cancer Discov.* **2021**, *2*, 568–576. [CrossRef] [PubMed]
25. Gagelmann, N.; Passamonti, F.; Wolschke, C.; Massoud, R.; Niederwieser, C.; Adjallé, R.; Mora, B.; Ayuk, F.; Kröger, N. Antibody response after vaccination against SARS-CoV-2 in adults with hematological malignancies: A systematic review and meta-analysis. *Haematologica* **2022**, *107*, 1840–1849. [CrossRef]
26. Fontana, L.M.; Villamagna, A.H.; Sikka, M.K.; McGregor, J.C. Understanding viral shedding of severe acute respiratory coronavirus virus 2 (SARS-CoV-2): Review of current literature. *Infect. Control Hosp. Epidemiol.* **2021**, *42*, 659–668. [CrossRef]

Disclaimer/Publisher's Note: The statements, opinions and data contained in all publications are solely those of the individual author(s) and contributor(s) and not of MDPI and/or the editor(s). MDPI and/or the editor(s) disclaim responsibility for any injury to people or property resulting from any ideas, methods, instructions or products referred to in the content.

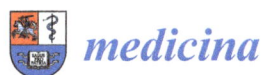

Case Report

A Cluster of Paragonimiasis with Delayed Diagnosis Due to Difficulty Distinguishing Symptoms from Post-COVID-19 Respiratory Symptoms: A Report of Five Cases

Jun Sasaki [1,*], Masanobu Matsuoka [1], Takashi Kinoshita [1], Takayuki Horii [1], Shingo Tsuneyoshi [1], Daiki Murata [1], Reiko Takaki [1], Masaki Tominaga [1], Mio Tanaka [2], Haruhiko Maruyama [2], Tomotaka Kawayama [1] and Tomoaki Hoshino [1]

[1] Department of Internal Medicine, Division of Respirology, Neurology, and Rheumatology, Kurume University School of Medicine, Kurume 830-0011, Japan
[2] Department of Infectious Diseases, Division of Parasitology, Faculty of Medicine, University of Miyazaki, Miyazaki 889-1692, Japan
* Correspondence: sasaki_jun@med.kurume-u.ac.jp; Tel.: +81-942-31-7560

Abstract: Paragonimiasis caused by trematodes belonging to the genus *Paragonimus* is often accompanied by chronic respiratory symptoms such as cough, the accumulation of sputum, hemoptysis, and chest pain. Prolonged symptoms, including respiratory symptoms, after coronavirus disease 2019 infection (COVID-19) are collectively called post-COVID-19 conditions. Paragonimiasis and COVID-19 may cause similar respiratory symptoms. We encountered five cases of paragonimiasis in patients in Japan for whom diagnoses were delayed due to the initial characterization of the respiratory symptoms as a post-COVID-19 condition. The patients had consumed homemade drunken freshwater crabs together. One to three weeks after consuming the crabs, four of the five patients were diagnosed with probable COVID-19. The major symptoms reported included cough, dyspnea, and chest pain. The major imaging findings were pleural effusion, pneumothorax, and nodular lesions of the lung. All the patients were diagnosed with paragonimiasis based on a serum antibody test and peripheral blood eosinophilia (560–15,610 cells/µL) and were treated successfully with 75 mg/kg/day praziquantel for 3 days. Before diagnosing a post-COVID-19 condition, it is necessary to consider whether other diseases, including paragonimiasis, may explain the symptoms. Further, chest radiographic or blood tests should be performed in patients with persistent respiratory symptoms after being infected with COVID-19 to avoid overlooking the possibility of infection.

Keywords: pulmonary paragonimiasis; *Paragonimus westermani*; COVID-19; post-COVID-19 condition; delayed diagnosis; case cluster

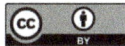

1. Introduction

Paragonimiasis is a food-borne parasitic disease caused by trematodes belonging to the genus *Paragonimus*, for which the majority are found in Asia. Humans can become infected by consuming raw or uncooked freshwater crabs, crayfish, or the meat of wild boars or deer. Although some cases are asymptomatic, the presenting symptoms typically include cough, the accumulation of sputum, and chest pain [1]. Delayed diagnosis has been reported due to the presence of atypical symptoms or an abnormal clinical course [2].

The coronavirus disease 2019 (COVID-19) pandemic has led to the delayed diagnosis of various diseases, including lung cancer [3], gynecological cancer [4], breast cancer [4,5], and gastrointestinal cancer [6]. COVID-19 can cause prolonged symptoms such as dyspnea and cough after infection, resulting in a post-COVID-19 condition [7]. As the number of post-acute COVID-19 patients has increased, so has the importance of excluding the possibility of other respiratory infections in individuals with persistent respiratory symptoms.

Herein, we report a cluster of five Japanese cases of paragonimiasis in which a diagnosis was delayed due to the mischaracterization of the symptoms as a post-COVID-19 condition.

2. Case Report

The clinical characteristics of the patients considered are summarized in Table 1. Of the patients, three were women and two were men, with a mean age of 39.2 years (range, 36–42 years). Cases 1 and 2 were housemates, and Cases 3 and 4 were a married couple. None of the patients had any relevant medical history, smoking history, or bronchial asthma. One patient (Case 4) had a history of allergic pollinosis.

Table 1. Clinical findings of the five cases considered.

	Case 1	Case 2	Case 3	Case 4	Case 5
Age (y), Sex	38, M	38, F	42, F	42, M	36, F
Symptoms					
Respiratory	Cough Dyspnea	Cough Dyspnea	Cough	Cough	Cough
Chest pain	+	+	−	−	−
Others	Fatigue	Epigastric pain	−	−	Abdominal discomfort
Radiographic and CT findings					
Intrapulmonary lesion	Nodular lesion	Infiltration	−	Nodular lesion	−
Pleural lesion	Pleural effusion	Pleural effusion Pneumothorax	Pleural effusion Pneumothorax	Pleural effusion Pneumothorax	Pleural effusion
Intraperitoneal lesion	Ascites	−	−	−	Linear low attenuation area of the liver
Peripheral blood					
WBC (cells/μL)	10,300	10,600	11,000	21,800	5700
Eosinophils (/μL)	5310	1290	5430	15,610	560
Eosinophil %	51.4%	12.2%	49.4%	71.5%	9.8%
IgE (IU/L)	1857	3487	96	2529	31
COVID-19 before diagnosis	Yes	Probably *	Yes	Probably *	No
Time from symptoms' onset to diagnosis (mos)	5	5	5	6	6
Treatment					
PZQ	+	+	+	+	+
Others	−	Drainage of pleural fluid	−	−	−

COVID-19, coronavirus disease 2019; CT, computed tomography; IgE, immunoglobulin E; PZQ, praziquantel; WBC, white blood cell count. * Patients had been in close contact with persons with COVID-19 without a confirmatory test.

All five patients consumed raw freshwater crabs (self-prepared drunken crabs) at a dinner party that they had attended together. One to three weeks after the party, four of the five patients presented to our hospital with complaints regarding a cough and were diagnosed with confirmed or likely COVID-19 (for two patients, this was confirmed by an antigen test). The mean time from the symptoms' onset to the initial visit to our hospital was 5.4 months.

Three patients presented to their primary care physicians complaining of respiratory symptoms before visiting our hospital. All three patients were considered to be affected by post-COVID-19 symptoms. Of the three patients, two were placed under observation and one (Case 1), who had asthma-like symptoms including a fluctuating cough and dyspnea, was treated with inhaled corticosteroids (ICS)/long-acting β_2 agonist (LABA) and 15 mg of oral prednisolone (PSL) for 3 weeks. The inhalation of ICS/LABA led to a temporary improvement in his symptoms.

At our hospital, the reported symptoms included cough (all patients), dyspnea (three patients), chest pain (two patients), fatigue (one patient), epigastric pain (one patient), and abdominal discomfort (one patient). Physical examination revealed a slight fever in Case 1 and bilateral decreases in breath sounds of the lower lung in Cases 1 and 4. Blood tests showed increased levels of eosinophils ranging from 560 to 15,610/µL (9.8–71.5%) in all five patients and increased levels of immunoglobulin E (IgE) ranging from 1857 to 3487 IU/L in three of the five patients. In contrast, C-reactive protein levels were near normal. Chest radiography and computed tomography (CT) showed pleural effusion (all patients), pneumothorax (three patients), nodular lesions with a cavity (one patient) and without cavity (one patient), infiltration of the lung (one patient), ascites (one patient), and a linear low attenuation area of the liver (one patient) (Figure 1A–E).

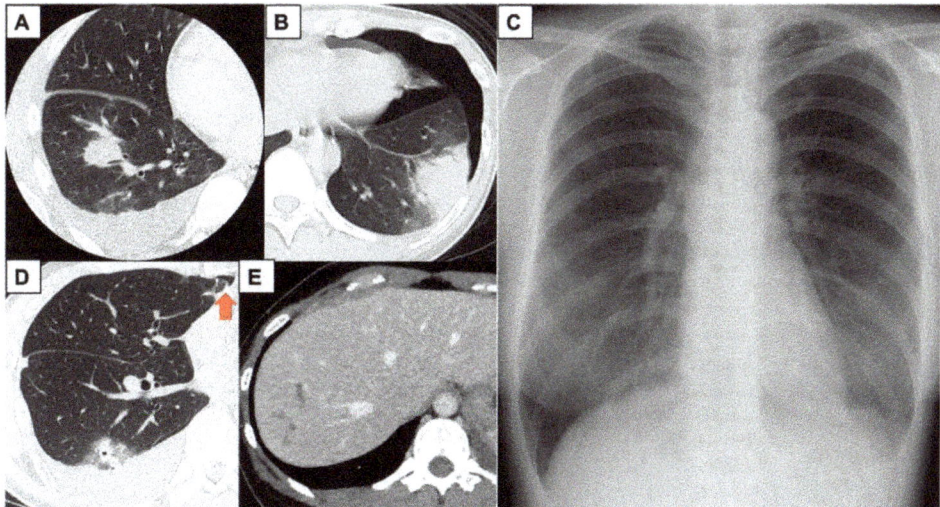

Figure 1. Imaging findings of cases. (**A**) Chest computed tomography (CT) of Case 1 showing a right-sided lung nodule and pleural effusion at the patient's initial visit; (**B**) chest CT of Case 2 showing left-sided infiltration of the lower lung and pneumothorax 2 months prior to visiting our hospital; (**C**) chest X-ray of Case 3 showing left pleural effusion and pneumothorax; (**D**) chest CT of Case 4 showing a right-sided lung nodule with cavity, pleural effusion, and pneumothorax (arrow); (**E**) contrast-enhanced abdominal CT of Case 5 showing a linear low attenuation area of the liver, likely representing a pathway for worm migration.

Pleural effusion fluid was examined in two patients. Both patients had exudative effusions, with a predominance of eosinophils and lymphocytes in Case 4 and lymphocytes in Case 5, examined by manual cell counting. A bronchoscopy was performed only in Case 1. To distinguish lung cancer and tuberculosis, a transbronchial lung biopsy of a right-sided nodule was performed. The biopsy specimen showed inflammatory changes, mainly eosinophils, without parasite eggs. Based on the finding of eosinophilia and the dietary history of raw freshwater crab consumption, we suggested that the symptoms were probably caused by a parasitic infection. We searched for parasite eggs in the pleural effusion and bronchial lavage fluid as well; however, we could not find any eggs. All five patients had high titers of serum *Paragonimus* IgG antibody, which was measured using a microplate enzyme-linked immunosorbent assay (ELISA). Cross-competition ELISA between *P. westermani* and *P. s. miyazakii* antigens suggested *P. westermani* infection.

All patients were treated with 75 mg/kg/day of praziquantel (PZQ) for 3 days, which led to an improvement in their symptoms and signs, including cough and dyspnea, eosinophilia, and pleural effusion. In Case 2, pleural fluid drainage was performed prior to PZQ administration.

3. Discussion

The incidence of paragonimiasis has decreased in Japan, and the number of cases diagnosed annually ranges from 17 to 49 [8]. Clustered or familial infections can occur [8,9]. According to a Japanese retrospective case review that considered 443 patients with paragonimiasis, the reported frequencies of symptoms were as follows: cough, 28.9%; sputum (including hemoptysis), 27.3%; chest pain, 18.5%; fever, 11.7%; dyspnea, 10.4%; and asymptomatic, 17.2% [1]. The most frequently observed finding on chest radiographs was pleural effusion (47.0%), followed by pneumothorax (16.9%), nodular shadows (11.5%), infiltrative shadows (8.8%), and mass shadows (6.5%) [1]. In the cases considered in this report, the symptoms and radiographic findings were consistent with those previously described. Furthermore, Case 5 appeared to have ectopic paragonimiasis in the liver.

A certain proportion of patients with COVID-19 experience sequelae after infection, which is known as long COVID [10] or post-acute COVID-19 syndrome [11]. The World Health Organization (WHO) has proposed that COVID-19-associated sequelae be referred to as a "post-COVID-19 condition" [7]. The prevalence of post-COVID-19 symptoms varies depending on the geographical area, survey method, and patient background. A Japanese cross-sectional study found the prevalence of cough, dyspnea, and chest pain to be 14.2%, 10.2%, and 2.4%, respectively (at a median duration of 29 days after the onset of COVID-19) [12]. The predominant CT pattern of COVID-19 revealed ground-glass opacity in the early stage and consolidation in later disease [13]. Pleural effusion and pneumothorax are uncommon in COVID-19 [14], a finding that differs from that of paragonimiasis. These findings were present in our patients.

In the cases considered in this study, the patients obtained freshwater crabs (the Japanese mitten crab) from a market. A meal of homemade drunken crabs was consumed by seven people. Six of the seven visited our hospital, with five suffering from paragonimiasis. Among the five patients with paragonimiasis, four had been previously diagnosed with or had been considered likely to be affected by COVID-19. Clearly, it was challenging for both patients and physicians to look past a diagnosis of a "post-COVID-19 condition". Atypical findings of eosinophilia, pleural effusion, and pneumothorax helped to exclude the possibility that the patients were afflicted by a post-COVID-19 condition, leading to the correct diagnosis of paragonimiasis. These cases highlight the importance of educating citizens regarding the safe preparation of freshwater crab. In addition, health centers should alert markets that sell infected freshwater crabs to any potential danger. Moreover, physicians should be aware they may encounter patients with paragonimiasis due to the globalization of dietary cultures.

In Case 1, the asthma-like symptoms of cough and dyspnea improved immediately after the inhalation of ICS/LABA and oral PSL, although the patient had no history of bronchial asthma or allergy. The effectiveness of ICS/LABA and PSL may contribute to the delayed diagnosis of paragonimiasis. Harada et al. [15] reported a case of bronchodilator reversibility in the acute phase of paragonimiasis. Jeon et al. [16] described bronchoscopic findings in 13 patients with paragonimiasis with intrapulmonary parenchymal lesions; in total, seven patients showed bronchial luminal narrowing and congested or edematous mucosal changes. Among the seven patients, bronchial mucosal biopsies revealed chronic inflammation with eosinophilic infiltrations in three patients. These findings are similar to those observed in patients with bronchial asthma. Dyspnea in patients with paragonimiasis might be caused by an asthma-like mechanism and not only by pleural effusion or pneumothorax.

4. Conclusions

In conclusion, physicians should consider whether diagnoses other than post-COVID-19 conditions such as paragonimiasis may explain respiratory symptoms in patients suspected to have recently been infected with COVID-19. Physicians should examine chest radiographs and blood tests in patients with persistent respiratory symptoms after COVID-19 to aid correct diagnoses.

Author Contributions: Conceptualization, M.M.; interpretation of imaging findings; T.H. (Takayuki Horii), S.T., D.M. and R.T.; provision of the patients' antibody test results, M.T. (Mio Tanaka) and H.M.; writing the manuscript, J.S.; editing of the manuscript, M.M., T.K. (Takashi Kinoshita), M.T. (Masaki Tominaga) and T.K. (Tomotaka Kawayama); supervision, T.H. (Tomoaki Hoshino). All authors have read and agreed to the published version of the manuscript.

Funding: This research received no external funding.

Institutional Review Board Statement: The study was conducted in accordance with the Declaration of Helsinki and approved by local ethics board of the Kurume University Hospital (protocol code, 2022-090; date of approval, 16 November 2022).

Informed Consent Statement: Informed consent for publication of their case details was obtained from all case patients described in this report.

Data Availability Statement: Data supporting the study findings are available from the corresponding author on reasonable request.

Conflicts of Interest: The authors declare no conflict of interest.

References

1. Nagayasu, E.; Yoshida, A.; Hombu, A.; Horii, Y.; Maruyama, H. Paragonimiasis in Japan: A twelve-year retrospective case review (2001–2012). *Intern. Med.* **2015**, *54*, 179–186. [CrossRef] [PubMed]
2. Kong, L.; Hua, L.; Liu, Q.; Bao, C.; Hu, J.; Xu, S. One delayed diagnosis of paragonimiasis case and literature review. *Respirol. Case Rep.* **2021**, *9*, e00750. [CrossRef] [PubMed]
3. Terashima, T.; Tsutsumi, A.; Iwami, E.; Kuroda, A.; Nakajima, T.; Eguchi, K. Delayed visit and treatment of lung cancer during the coronavirus disease 2019 pandemic in Japan: A retrospective study. *J. Int. Med. Res.* **2022**, *50*, 3000605221097375. [CrossRef] [PubMed]
4. Knoll, K.; Reiser, E.; Leitner, K.; Kogl, J.; Ebner, C.; Marth, C.; Tsibulak, I. The impact of COVID-19 pandemic on the rate of newly diagnosed gynecological and breast cancers: A tertiary center perspective. *Arch. Gynecol. Obstet.* **2022**, *305*, 945–953. [CrossRef] [PubMed]
5. Linck, P.A.; Garnier, C.; Depetiteville, M.P.; MacGrogan, G.; Mathoulin-Pelissier, S.; Quenel-Tueux, N.; Charitansky, H.; Boisserie-Lacroix, M.; Chamming's, F. Impact of the COVID-19 lockdown in France on the diagnosis and staging of breast cancers in a tertiary cancer center. *Eur. Radiol.* **2022**, *32*, 1644–1651. [CrossRef] [PubMed]
6. Kuzuu, K.; Misawa, N.; Ashikari, K.; Kessoku, T.; Kato, S.; Hosono, K.; Yoneda, M.; Nonaka, T.; Matsushima, S.; Komatsu, T.; et al. Gastrointestinal cancer stage at diagnosis before and during the COVID-19 pandemic in Japan. *JAMA Netw. Open* **2021**, *4*, e2126334. [CrossRef] [PubMed]
7. Soriano, J.B.; Murthy, S.; Marshall, J.C.; Relan, P.; Diaz, J.V. WHO Clinical Case Definition Working Group on Post-COVID-19 Condition. A clinical case definition of post-COVID-19 condition by a Delphi consensus. *Lancet Infect. Dis.* **2022**, *22*, e102–e107. [CrossRef] [PubMed]
8. Yoshida, A.; Doanh, P.N.; Maruyama, H. Paragonimus and paragonimiasis in Asia: An update. *Acta Trop.* **2019**, *199*, 105074. [CrossRef]
9. Sohn, B.S.; Bae, Y.J.; Cho, Y.S.; Moon, H.B.; Kim, T.B. Three cases of paragonimiasis in a family. *Korean J. Parasitol.* **2009**, *47*, 281–285. [CrossRef]
10. Sudre, C.H.; Murray, B.; Varsavsky, T.; Graham, M.S.; Penfold, R.S.; Bowyer, R.C.; Pujol, J.C.; Klaser, K.; Antonelli, M.; Canas, L.S.; et al. Attributes and predictors of long COVID. *Nat. Med.* **2021**, *27*, 626–631. [CrossRef] [PubMed]
11. Nalbandian, A.; Sehgal, K.; Gupta, A.; Madhavan, M.V.; McGroder, C.; Stevens, J.S.; Cook, J.R.; Nordvig, A.S.; Shalev, D.; Sehrawat, T.S.; et al. Post-acute COVID-19 syndrome. *Nat. Med.* **2021**, *27*, 601–615. [CrossRef] [PubMed]
12. Sugiyama, A.; Miwata, K.; Kitahara, Y.; Okimoto, M.; Abe, K.; Ouoba, S.; Akita, T.; Tanimine, N.; Ohdan, H.; Kubo, T.; et al. Long COVID occurrence in COVID-19 survivors. *Sci. Rep.* **2022**, *12*, 6039. [CrossRef] [PubMed]
13. Fischer, T.; El Baz, Y.; Scanferla, G.; Graf, N.; Waldeck, F.; Kleger, G.R.; Frauenfelder, T.; Bremerich, J.; Kobbe, S.S.; Pagani, J.L.; et al. Comparison of temporal evolution of computed tomography imaging features in COVID-19 and influenza infections in a multicenter cohort study. *Eur. J. Radiol. Open* **2022**, *9*, 100431. [CrossRef] [PubMed]

14. Salehi, S.; Abedi, A.; Balakrishnan, S.; Gholamrezanezhad, A. Coronavirus disease 2019 (COVID-19): A systematic review of imaging findings in 919 patients. *AJR Am. J. Roentgenol.* **2020**, *215*, 87–93. [CrossRef] [PubMed]
15. Harada, T.; Kawasaki, Y.; Tsukada, A.; Osawa, Y.; Takami, H.; Yamaguchi, K.; Kurai, J.; Yamasaki, A.; Shimizu, E. Bronchodilator reversibility occurring during the acute phase of paragonimiasis westermani infection. *Intern. Med.* **2019**, *58*, 297–300. [CrossRef] [PubMed]
16. Jeon, K.; Koh, W.J.; Kim, H.; Kwon, O.J.; Kim, T.S.; Lee, K.S.; Han, J. Clinical features of recently diagnosed pulmonary paragonimiasis in Korea. *Chest* **2005**, *128*, 1423–1430. [CrossRef] [PubMed]

Disclaimer/Publisher's Note: The statements, opinions and data contained in all publications are solely those of the individual author(s) and contributor(s) and not of MDPI and/or the editor(s). MDPI and/or the editor(s) disclaim responsibility for any injury to people or property resulting from any ideas, methods, instructions or products referred to in the content.

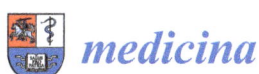

Article

Lung Ultrasound Is Useful for Evaluating Lung Damage in COVID-19 Patients Treated with Bamlanivimab and Etesevimab: A Single-Center Pilot Study

Sebastiano Cicco [1], Marialuisa Sveva Marozzi [1], Carmen Alessandra Palumbo [1], Elisabetta Sturdà [1], Antonio Fusillo [1], Flavio Scarilli [1], Federica Albanese [1], Claudia Morelli [1], Davide Fiore Bavaro [2], Lucia Diella [2], Annalisa Saracino [2], Fabrizio Pappagallo [1], Antonio Giovanni Solimando [1,*], Gianfranco Lauletta [1], Roberto Ria [1] and Angelo Vacca [1]

[1] COVID Section, Unit of Internal Medicine "Guido Baccelli", Department of Precision and Regenerative Medicine and Ionian Area (DiMePre-J), University of Bari Aldo Moro, I-70124 Bari, Italy
[2] Unit of Infectious Diseases, Department of Precision and Regenerative Medicine and Ionian Area (DiMePre-J), University of Bari Aldo Moro, I-70124 Bari, Italy
* Correspondence: antonio.solimando@uniba.it

Abstract: *Background and Objectives:* COVID-19 induces massive systemic inflammation. Researchers have spent much time and effort finding an excellent and rapid image tool to evaluate COVID-19 patients. Since the pandemic's beginning, lung ultrasound (LUS) has been identified for this purpose. Monoclonal antibodies (mAb) were used to treat mild patients and prevent respiratory disease worsening. *Materials and Methods:* We evaluated 15 Caucasian patients with mild COVID-19 who did not require home oxygen, treated with Bamlanivimab and Etesevimab (Group 1). A molecular nose–throat swab test confirmed the diagnosis. All were office patients, and nobody was affected by respiratory failure. They were admitted to receive the single-day infusion of mAb treatment in agreement with the Italian Drug Agency (AIFA) rules for approval. LUS was performed before the drug administration (T0) and after three months (T1). We compared LUS at T1 in other outpatients who came for follow-up and were overlapping at the time of diagnosis for admittance criteria to receive mAb (Group 2). *Results:* Our COVID-19 outpatients reported no hospitalization in a follow-up visit after recovery. All patients became SARS-CoV-2 negative within one month since T0. LUS score at T0 was 8.23 ± 6.46. At T1 we found a significant decrease in Group 1 LUS score (5.18 ± 4.74; $p < 0.05$). We also found a significant decrease in the LUS score of Group 1 T1 compared to Group2 T1 (5.18 ± 4.74 vs 7.82 ± 5.21; $p < 0.05$). *Conclusion:* Early treatment of the SARS-CoV-2 virus effectively achieves a better recovery from disease and reduces lung involvement after three months as evaluated with LUS. Despite extrapolation to the general population may be done with caution, based on our data this ultrasound method is also effective for evaluating and following lung involvement in COVID-19 patients.

Keywords: Bamlanivimab; Etesevimab; COVID-19; lung ultrasound

Citation: Cicco, S.; Marozzi, M.S.; Palumbo, C.A.; Sturdà, E.; Fusillo, A.; Scarilli, F.; Albanese, F.; Morelli, C.; Bavaro, D.F.; Diella, L.; et al. Lung Ultrasound Is Useful for Evaluating Lung Damage in COVID-19 Patients Treated with Bamlanivimab and Etesevimab: A Single-Center Pilot Study. *Medicina* 2023, 59, 203. https://doi.org/10.3390/medicina59020203

Academic Editor: Masaki Okamoto

Received: 7 December 2022
Revised: 13 January 2023
Accepted: 16 January 2023
Published: 19 January 2023

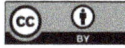

Copyright: © 2023 by the authors. Licensee MDPI, Basel, Switzerland. This article is an open access article distributed under the terms and conditions of the Creative Commons Attribution (CC BY) license (https://creativecommons.org/licenses/by/4.0/).

1. Introduction

The coronavirus disease 2019 (COVID-19) continues to exert an enormous global public health impact. The SARS-CoV-2 infection induces a robust systemic inflammation that presents an extensive range of symptoms from mild to severe. A high death rate has been reported in a vulnerable subgroup of patients [1]. The risk of death increases among older patients and those with chronic medical conditions such as cardiovascular disease, diabetes, obesity, lung disease, and cancer [2]. The more common symptoms are dyspnea, fatigue, fever, malaise, and anosmia. The disease may progress to more severe complications, including pneumonia and acute respiratory distress syndrome [3]. Researchers have spent time and effort finding a valuable and easy tool to evaluate these patients [4].

Due to the specific aspects of the infection, which mainly begins in the peripheral lung parenchyma, lung ultrasonography (LUS) is suitable as a diagnostic imaging method to identify suspected cases in the early disease phases [5]. LUS was identified for this purpose since the pandemic's beginning. Serial ultrasound examinations on patients with confirmed COVID-19 can promptly detect changes in the affected lung tissue [5,6]. Moreover, many resources have been used to identify an adequate and effective treatment. One approach is neutralizing monoclonal antibodies (mAb). Bamlanivimab and Etesevimab neutralize immunoglobulin G (IgG)-1 mAb directed to the receptor-binding domain (RBD) of the spike (S) protein of SARS-CoV-2 [4]. Both mAb in combination were the first mAb therapy used to treat mild COVID-19 patients to prevent the worsening of respiratory disease. We studied LUS in COVID-19 patients treated with Bamlanivimab and Etesevimab and evaluated its changes after treatment and whether these were related to disease recovery. We compared the clinical outcomes of a control group treated at home without mAb.

2. Materials and Methods

2.1. Study Population

This study represented a pilot subgroup analysis of a more extensive study performed at our institution [7]. The primary study was approved by the Ethics Committee of the University of Bari Medical School [n° 6357/2020], and it conformed to the good clinical practice guidelines of the Italian Ministry of Health and the ethical guidelines of the Declaration of Helsinki, as revised and amended in 2004. To avoid possible clinical confounders, patients with already known interstitial lung disease were excluded. We evaluated 15 Caucasian patients (9 males and 6 females, aged 64.50 ± 7.26, Group 1) whose nose–throat swab test results were positive between March and April 2021 (third COVID-19 wave in Italy) with mild COVID-19 disease that did not require home oxygen treatment at the time of enrolment. A molecular nose–throat swab test confirmed the diagnosis within 7 days, with less than 10 days of COVID-19 symptoms. Patients were admitted as outpatients, had oxygen saturation higher than 92%, and nobody was affected by respiratory failure. The patients received Bamlanivimab and Etesevimab as a single-day infusion treatment to prevent further COVID-19 disease evolution. Admission for the mAb treatment was performed in accordance with the Italian Drug Agency (AIFA) at the time of approval for treatment [8]. Each patient was evaluated before the drug was given (T0) and after three months (T1). We had the check after three months, as suggested by the Apulian Healthcare system as a standard follow-up time-point. As a control group, we evaluated 28 patients (16 males and 12 females, aged 59.71 ± 11.68, Group 2), as outpatients admitted to our post-COVID-19 office for the follow-up of residual lung disease three months after recovery of the disease (T1). No one in either group was vaccinated against COVID-19. They were not hospitalized and were comparable for admittance criteria to be treated with mAb. They experienced the SARS-CoV-2 disease in the same period as Group 1. They were treated with antibiotics, anti-inflammatories, and/or corticosteroids, but not with mAb. They were not evaluated at the onset of disease (T0) because according to the standard of care protocol of the Apulian Health Care System, the first evaluation was performed at home by other physicians; hence, no data were available about medical examination and LUS. Thus, we compared Group 1 to Group 2 only at T1.

2.2. Study Protocol

General practitioners indicated that patients affected by COVID-19 should be elective for mAb treatment via a dedicated service. All patients underwent a complete history collection the afternoon before administration to check their clinical status and eligibility via a telemedicine consult. At T0, patients were managed by the hospital's outpatient service according to the local guidelines [7]. The patients underwent a complete physical examination and blood pressure measurement. A good practice is the evaluation of SpO_2 before administration of mAb: 94% is the cut-off to consider a respiratory involvement severity [8]. We evaluated blood gas analysis to be more on-target and administered mAb in patients who may have benefitted according to clinical trials [9]. Blood gas analysis was performed on an arterial blood sample to evaluate oxygen (pO2), carbon dioxide (pCO2), oxygen saturation percentage (sO2), blood HCO_3^-, and pH. The ratio between the oxygen of the inspired fraction (P/F ratio) and the arterial–alveolar oxygen difference (A-aDO2) was also measured. The infusion was administered as scheduled [10]. Next, the patients were observed for one hour to rule out early drug reactions. The patients' follow-up was via phone call, and they came as outpatients after three months (T1). In both Group 1 and Group 2, a daily body temperature and as standardized measurements, the mean temperature between day 7 and day 10 were recorded. Nasopharyngeal (NP) SARS-CoV-2 RNA swabs were collected every 7 days from the first positive one. Recovery was defined when the first negative NP swab was detected. At the office T1 evaluation, patients performed spirometry next to a new lung ultrasound and blood gas analysis.

2.3. Lung Ultrasound

This was performed after patients rested for 10 min in a sitting position. A 5–12 MHz ultrasound probe was used. Depth was 10 cm with a focus on the pleural line. LUS was performed before the drug was given (T0) and after three months (T1). According to the international guideline indications [6,11] the LUS was evaluated on six segments for each lung, and each segment was scored as 0 for less than 3 B-lines, 1 for more than 3 B-lines, 2 for B-lines more than 50%, and 3 for white lung or consolidation (Figure 1). The same operator performed all LUS. The operator was blinded on the comorbidities. A second expert operator validated the LUS score evaluation, blinded from the first evaluation. In disagreement, a third expert (C.M.) evaluation was considered a referral.

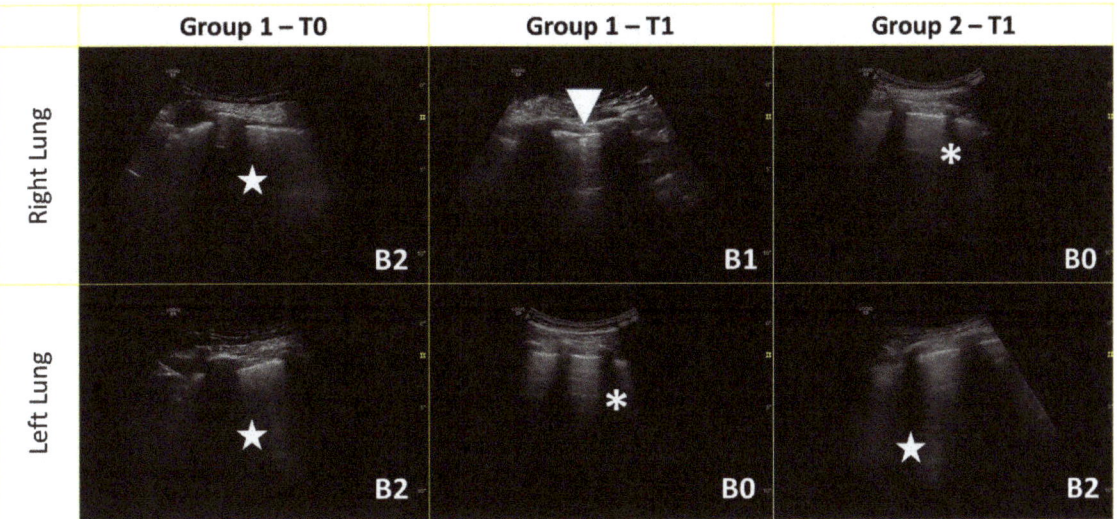

Figure 1. Representative images from one patient for each group (at the different time points) from the right and left lungs used to evaluate the lung ultrasound (LUS) score. The score for each segment is reported at the bottom of each panel. Multiple B-line conglomerations are indicated with (★), B-lines with little subpleural consolidation are indicated with (▼) while (✱) indicates A-lines.

2.4. Statistics

Data were analyzed using GraphPad Prism software (La Jolla, CA, USA) and expressed as means ± S.D. for parametric data and median and interquartile range (IQR). The distribution of dichotomous values was analyzed with the Chi-square test. Regarding non-normally distributed data, we performed a non-parametric Mann–Whitney test for comparisons and Spearman distribution for correlations. Normally distributed data were studied with a parametric unpaired t-test for comparisons and Pearson distribution for correlation. Statistical significance was indicated with a value of $p < 0.05$. To understand if the LUS score in Group 1 related to clinical features, a regression was performed with clinical symptoms, blood pressure, heart rate, respiratory rate, temperature, and with blood gas analysis results.

3. Results

3.1. Population Differences

We evaluated two groups of Caucasian patients. Group 1 was composed of 15 patients with mild COVID-19 disease treated with Bamlanivimab and Etesevimab mAb; Group 2 was composed of 28 patients with mild COVID-19 disease treated at home with canonical drugs but not with mAb. The groups were comparable for age and sex, comorbidities, and risk factors, as shown in Table 1. Group 1 patients presented the same distribution of comorbidities as Group 2, but had significantly increased BMI (Table 1).

Table 1. Clinical features of Group 1 (mAb) and Group 2 (no mAb) patients.

	mAb	No mAb	p-Value
Age	64.50 ± 7.26	59.71 ± 11.68	Ns
Sex (M/F)	8/6	16/12	Ns
Body mass index (kg/m^2)	34.70 ± 3.07	26.48 ± 1.57	0.0001
Comorbidities number (IQR)	2 (–2.5)	1 (1.2)	Ns
Diabetes	2	2	Ns
Arterial hypertension	10	15	Ns
Cardiovascular disease	7	4	Ns
Chronic obstructive pulmonary disease	4	3	Ns
Other lung diseases (Asthma, Obstructive sleep apnea)	1	2	Ns
Chronic kidney disease	1	0	Ns
Chronic liver disease	1	0	Ns
Autoimmune disease	1	4	Ns
Cancer	2	3	Ns
Current Smoker	2	4	Ns

COVID: Coronavirus Disease; IQR: interquartile range.

3.2. mAb role in COVID-19 Recovery

Group 1 and Group 2 patients presented the same number of symptoms. However, Group 1 showed a significant decrease in mean temperature on days 7 to 10 compared to Group 2 (Table 2). Patients in Group 2 presented an increased max temperature during COVID disease compared to Group 1 (Group 1 37.06 ± 0.98 vs. Group 1 38.66 ± 0.52 °C, $p = 0.0001$). Patients in Group 1 presented with fewer symptoms reported compared to Group 2, but this result showed a statistical tendency ($p = 0.05$) to significance (Table 2). Moreover, cough, myalgia, and fatigue were mostly reported, but no difference was found in the number for each single symptom between the groups (Table 2). However, the main difference between the groups concerned the time to recovery. As shown in Table 2, in both groups, the majority of patients became SARS-CoV-2 negative within the first month of treatment. However, the infusion of Bamlanivimab and Etesevimab shortened symptom duration and reduced the time of NP SARS-CoV-2 RNA negativization (Time of recovery: Group 1, 13.85 ± 7.91; Group 2, 21.65 ± 7.08, $p = 0.0007$) (Table 2). Similarly, a more significant number of patients recovered within 14 days in Group 1, whereas in Group 2 patients recovered within 28 days (Table 2).

Table 2. Group 1 (mAb) and Group 2 (no mAb) clinical features of the COVID-19 disease during the entire period of the illness.

	mAb	No mAb	
Time of recovery (first negative swab)	13.85 ± 7.91	21.65 ± 7.08	0.0007
14-day recovery (%)	10 (71.43)	2 (7.14)	<0.0001
28-day recovery (%)	12 (85.71)	21 (75.00)	Ns
Home-treated number (steroids, NSAIDs, paracetamol, prophylactic antibiotic)	9	18	Ns
Need of Oxygen (%)	2 (14.29)	1 (3.57)	Ns
Steroid (Prednisone)	3	9	Ns
Antibiotics	6	10	Ns
Low molecular weight heparin	3	1	Ns
COVID Symptoms median number (IQR)	3 (2–4)	4 (3–7)	0.05
Fever	7	22	Ns
Max Temperature	37.06 ± 0.98	38.66 ± 0.52	0.0001
Cough	12	26	Ns
Dyspnea	2	12	Ns
Tachypnea (>22 arpm)	0	6	Ns
Fatigue	5	13	Ns
Hypo/anosmia	3	14	Ns
Dysgeusia	4	14	Ns
Sore Throat	4	7	Ns
Nausea/vomiting	0	3	Ns
Diarrhea	2	7	Ns
Myalgia/arthralgia	7	9	Ns
Confusion	0	1	Ns
Headache	2	9	Ns
Conjunctivitis	0	2	Ns

COVID: Coronavirus Disease; IQR: interquartile range.

Bamlanivimab and Etesevimab were safe, and no side effects were observed. Only one patient was hospitalized after treatment for arrhythmia and heart failure. Nonetheless, based on clinically judged previous conditions, these symptoms were not related to COVID-19 lung disease or drug side effects related to mAb administration but rather to a volume overload.

3.3. Clinical Outcome

At T1 in Group 1, we found a decrease for both systolic (128.00 ± 15.67, vs. T0 146.90 ± 15.18, $p = 0.04$) and diastolic (71.00 ± 7.75 vs. T0 81.30 ± 7.62, $p = 0.03$) blood pressure (Table 3). At T1, systolic blood pressure did not differ between Group 1 and Group 2, while diastolic pressure was decreased in Group 1 (71.00 ± 7.75 vs. 81.67 ± 9.31 Group 2, $p = 0.03$) (Table 3). As expected, Group 1 showed a reduction in body temperature at T1 (35.87 ± 0.42) compared to T0 (37.06 ± 0.98, $p = 0.001$) (Table 3). Likewise, we performed the same analysis at T1 for Group 2.

Table 3. Group 1 (mAb) and Group 2 (No mAb) vital signs and blood gas analysis at diagnosis of SARS-CoV-2 infection (T0) and after 3 months (T1).

	mAb			No mAb	*p*-Value
	T0	T1	*p*-Value vs T0		*p*-Value vs T1
	Vital Signs				
Systolic blood pressure (mmHg)	146.90 ± 15.18	128.00 ± 15.67	0.04	127.50 ± 7.58	Ns
Diastolic blood pressure (mmHg)	81.30 ± 7.62	71.00 ± 7.75	0.03	81.67 ± 9.31	0.03
Heart rate (bpm)	74.57 ± 13.67	86.00 ± 13.70	Ns	78.86 ± 8.21	Ns
Respiration rate (apm)	19.33 ± 2.45	18.67 ± 2.00	Ns	16.00 ± 2.83	Ns
Temperature (°C)	37.06 ± 0.98	35.87 ± 0.42	0.001	-	
	Blood Gas Analysis				
pH	7.45 ± 0.03	7.42 ± 0.03	0.01	7.46 ± 0.05	0.04
pCO2 (mmHg)	37.91 ± 4.11	37.27 ± 2.97	ns	40.50 ± 1.29	0.03
pO2 (mmHg)	76.09 ± 11.84	88.27 ± 10.25	0.008	75.00 ± 9.83	0.04
HCO_3^- (mEq/L)	26.89 ± 2.34	24.81 ± 1.76	0.02	28.38 ± 3.13	0.01
SO_2 (%)	96.69 ± 1.84	98.08 ± 0.76	0.02	95.25 ± 2.36	0.004
A-aDO2 (mmHg)	26.52 ± 13.76	15.14 ± 9.74	0.02	24.38 ± 10.84	0.02
P/F	362.40 ± 56.22	420.30 ± 48.76	0.005	357.00 ± 46.72	0.04

A-aDO2: difference in Oxygen pressure between alveoli and arterial; Apm: acts per minute; bpm: beat per minute; HCO^{3-}: bicarbonate ion; mmHg: mercury millimeter; P/F: the ratio between pO2 and oxygen given (FiO$_2$); pCO2: arterial carbodioxyde partial pressure; pO2: arterial oxygen partial pressure; SO_2: oxygen saturation percentage; COVID: Coronavirus Disease; IQR: interquartile range.

There were great odds between blood gas analyses of the two groups. First, in Group 1, we found an improvement in gas exchange at T1 compared to T0: a significant increase in pO2 (88.27 ± 10.25 vs. 76.09 ± 11.84, $p = 0.008$) and in sO2 (98.08 ± 0.76 vs. 96.69 ± 1.84, $p = 0.02$); a significant decrease in A-aDO2 (15.14 ± 9.74 vs. 26.52 ± 13.76, $p = 0.02$) and increase in P/F ratio (420.30 ± 48.76 vs. 362.40 ± 56.22, $p = 0.005$) (Table 3). Finally, the HCO_3^- significantly decreased (24.81 ± 1.76 vs. 26.89 ± 4.11, $p = 0.02$) although pCO2 did not change, resulting in a decrease in pH (7.42 ± 0.03 vs. 7.45 ± 0.03, $p = 0.01$) (Table 3). In sum, Group 1 at T1 showed a complete recovery of respiratory function. In contrast, at T1, the blood gas analysis of the Group 2 overlapped that of Group 1 at T0. Group 2 displayed a significant decrease in pO2 (75.00 ± 9.83 vs. 88.27 ± 10.25, $p = 0.04$) and sO2 (95.25 ± 2.36 vs. 98.08 ± 0.76, $p = 0.004$) (Table 3). Similarly, Group 2 presented a significant increase in A-aDO2 (24.38 ± 10.84 vs. 15.14 ± 9.74, $p = 0.02$) and a decrease in P/F ratio (357.00 ± 46.72 vs. 420.30 ± 48.76, $p = 0.04$) (Table 3). Spirometry evaluation at T1 results were mostly normal, and there were no differences between the two groups (Supplementary Table S1).

3.4. Lung Ultrasound Score Evaluation

In Group 1, LUS at T1 decreased significantly compared to T0 (5.18 ± 4.74 vs. 8.23 ± 6.28; $p < 0.05$) (Figure 2). In particular, it reduced in 86.7% of patients (Supplementary Figure S1) while the results were stable in the remaining two. These patients presented diffuse lung involvement, especially in basal segments, ranging from a few B-lines to consolidations (pattern B3). At T1 we found a reduction in lung involvement, but the same increase in damage from the apex to the base was detected (Supplementary Table S4). At T1, the LUS was also significantly lower (7.82 ± 5.21; $p < 0.05$) in Group 1 compared to Group 2 (Figures 1 and 2). The LUS at T0 relates significantly to recovery days (Supplementary Table S3). Similarly, these results were found for LUS score at T1. It was significantly related to the length of disease evaluated as days to achieve swab recovery (Figure 3a—Supplementary Table S4). This result was not found in patients who did not experience mAb (Figure 3b—Supplementary Table S4). In Group 1, we did not find any correlation between LUS score and symptoms. LUS score relates directly to pH ($p = 0.013$), A-aDO2 ($p = 0.002$), heart rate ($p = 0.013$) and respiratory rate ($p = 0.021$) at T0. No other correlation was found and no correlation between LUS score and such parameters at T1 in Group 1 and in Group 2.

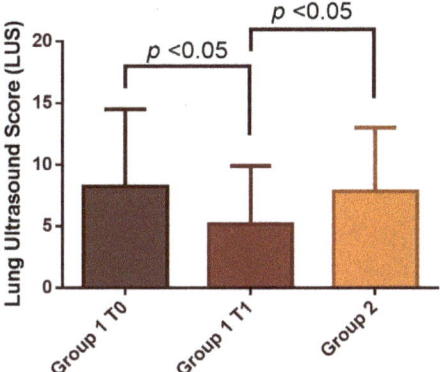

Figure 2. LUS score at the time of administration of mAb (T0) and at the 3-month visit (T1) compared to the LUS score found in the 3-month visit in patients who did not experience the mAb treatment.

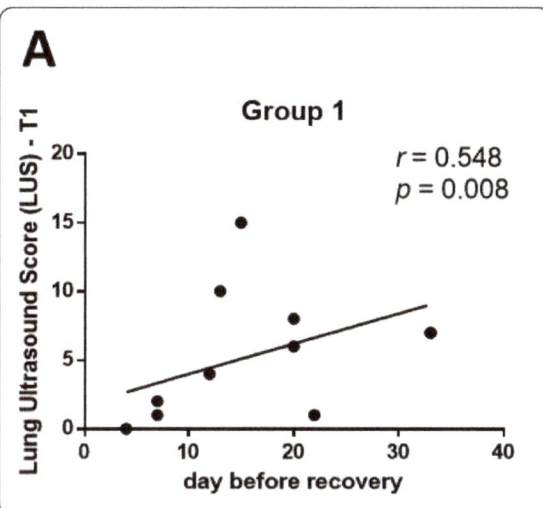
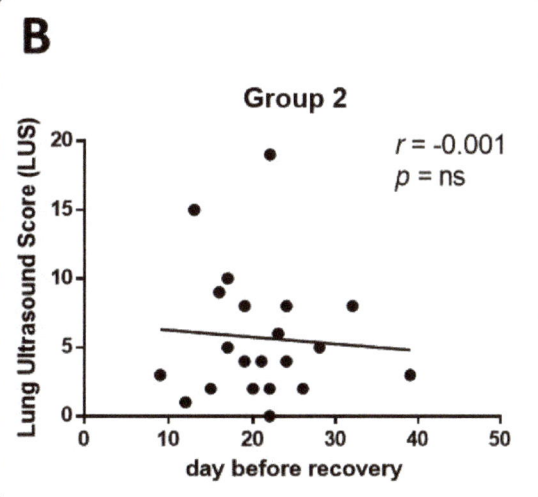

Figure 3. Correlation between the LUS scores evaluated at the follow-up visit and the days before recovery in patients who underwent mAb treatment and those who did not. (Panel (**A**)): correlation in Group 1 at T1 time point (follow-up visit). (Panel (**B**)): correlation in Group 2 at follow-up visit.

At T0, considering the blood gas analysis of lung involvement, we considered length (day) of recovery as the dependent variable. We found a significant correlation only to A-aDO2 in group 1 (Supplementary Table S3). A similar result was found in correlation between LUS at T0 and day before recovery (Supplementary Table S3). No correlation was found between blood gas analysis results and clinical symptoms recorded. At T1, the follow-up visit after recovery, length (day) of recovery was considered as an independent variable. We found a correlation to A-aDO2 only in Group 1 but not in Group 2 (Supplementary Table S4).

4. Discussion

Many efforts have been invested in improving the patients' care for the new COVID-19 pandemic [12–15]. The mAbs were the first specific treatment option to face this disease [16,17]. SARS-COV-2 enters cells after binding its spike protein to receptors for angiotensin-converting enzyme 2 (ACE2). This is particularly important considering the increased risk for patients with high cardiovascular risk [18,19]. Bamlanivimab is a mAb mimicking an anti-spike neutralizing antibody derived from convalescing COVID-19 patients. Bamlanivimab reduced viral replication by 10^2–10^5 in bronchoalveolar lavage on days 1, 3, and 6, and limited the respiratory and clinical signs of the disease [16]. Etesevimab has a similar structure and effectively reduced the viral load in a Rhesus monkey model of COVID-19 [17]. Bamlanivimab and Etesevimab bind to different epitopes of the receptor for ACE2.

The primary clinical use of Bamlanivimab and Etesevimab is to prevent hospitalizations and deaths. Their role in other outcomes, including longer-term ones, is still being determined. To our knowledge, no data on anti-COVID-19-specific mAb in lung recovery have been published so far. In addition, results on the lung recovery after modulation of inflammation using anti-cytokine mAb such as Tocilizumab are circumstantial [20–22].

Combined Bamlanivimab and Etesevimab treatment is safe [7] and given with the outpatient regimen, avoids the costs of hospitalizations. Using Bamlanivimab plus Etesevimab instead of Bamlanivimab alone did not lead to a significant difference in viral load reduction [9]. However, the early treatment effectively achieved better disease recovery. Moreover, patients with immune dysregulation well tolerated and benefited from these mAb [16]. Contrariwise mutation in the SARS-CoV-2 spike protein could invalidate the quick healing of the symptoms. However, no worsening of the status was observed, and chest X-ray and biological inflammatory markers usually persist [23]. Our patients did not develop adverse reactions and achieved an earlier recovery despite the fact that they were affected by several comorbidities (obesity, diabetes mellitus, renal failure, cardiovascular disease, lung disease, cirrhosis, immunosuppression condition, cancer).

Lung damage may also occur in asymptomatic/mild disease [24,25] and may persist in subsequent months [26–28]. Based on this literature and our data, the LUS and LUS score evaluation suggests that the combined Bamlanivimab and Etesevimab treatment could reduce lung involvement after three months. This ultrasound method has primarily been used during the pandemic to manage lung injury. It has high diagnostic accuracy compared with auscultation or radiographic imaging and can also be practiced on moderate, severe, and critical COVID-19-associated dyspnea [29]. It is also effective for evaluating and following lung involvement in COVID-19 patients. Our data suggest that mAb treatment improved vital signs after 3 months of recovery. This result may not have been a direct effect of treatment. Indeed, since COVID-19 affects the vascular endothelium [6,30,31], reducing the viral load by mAb may produce reduced vascular inflammation in the body, including the lungs.

Our data also indicate a good perspective for obese patients because some patients had higher body mass indexes. Obesity leads to increased inflammation leading to multiple related diseases [32–34]. In this view, COVID-19 represents another stimulus on top of the release of the cytokines described in obesity [35]. Thus, immunotherapy focused on inflammatory cytokine neutralization, immunomodulation, and passive viral neutralization may decrease inflammation, inflammation-associated lung injury, or viral load, and can also avoid acute hospitalization and mechanical ventilation dependency, all of which are restricted options.

Chen P et al. [36] showed that subjects who received a placebo gave a 6.3% incidence of admission to the hospital or emergency room compared to only 1.6% of those treated with Bamlavinivimab. Subsequently, in a phase 3 study, adults with a high risk of progressing to disease and at least one risk factor for the severe disease were tested. These patients were in early disease, i.e., within 3 days of diagnosis, and again, as outpatients. Compared to the placebo, there was a 70% risk reduction in the hospitalized individuals who received the Bamlanivimab and Etesevimab mAb. Thus, 7% of patients needed to be hospitalized in the placebo group compared to only 2.1% in the treatment one [4]. While confirming these data, we substantially extended these findings by providing a deeper insight into the real-life experience of the mAb-based treatment of COVID-19.

Limitations

This study had clear limitations. First, it was a single-center study, and we enrolled a relatively small sample size. Secondly, due to regional protocols for pandemic containment, the T0 evaluation needs to be improved in patients who were not treated with mAbs. However, based on the literature data [24–28], lung damage also occurs in asymptomatic or mild diseases. These patients are not treated with specific drugs; sequelae are detectable in subsequent follow-ups. Thirdly, given the lack of powered sample size, our findings need to be confirmed on a larger scale. Furthermore, our findings may be relevant in the context of the high incidence of variants of concern but may be less generalizable in other epidemiological settings. The knowledge of SARS-CoV-2 variants before mAb infusion is not feasible.

Moreover, since this was an observational (non-randomized) study, the choice to administer Bamlanivimab/Etesevimab was made according to drug availability and the prescriber's judgment and not to patients' clinical conditions, leading to a selection bias. Finally, it presents a real-life experience in fighting COVID-19 since there was no guideline on patients' treatment at the time of enrollment, so there was no standardization of the treatment. Therefore, concomitant treatments were not standardized. However, our data effectively suggest a role in early recovery for mAb treatment both as clinical and instrumental findings. Thus, it is tempting to use early treatment in COVID-19, especially in a LUS-guided approach. Our data demonstrate the role of early treatment in reducing lung damage. A working hypothesis may be using portable ultrasound equipment to have in-home monitoring for patients who experience early treatment (both antiviral or mAb) to have a tailored treatment and diagnosis. This may be useful to prevent vascular damage in long-term COVID-19 survivals. The decrease in diastolic blood pressure in patients who experienced mAb at T1 may suggest this hypothesis.

5. Conclusions

Lung ultrasound results effectively evaluated lung damage in patients who experienced monoclonal antibodies against COVID-19. In our little experience, the infusion of Bamlanivimab and Etesevimab shortened symptom duration and reduced the time of NP SARS-CoV-2 RNA negativization. In reference to its extrapolation to the general population, LUS with LUS score evaluation before and after recovery suggested that this treatment may reduce lung involvement. However, larger and more prospective studies are needed.

Supplementary Materials: The following supporting information can be downloaded at: https://www.mdpi.com/article/10.3390/medicina59020203/s1, Table S1: comparison between spirometry results between the two groups studied at T; Table S2: segment evaluation for each patient in Group 1 population as T0 and T1; Table S3: Day of recovery (evaluated as dependent variable), relates differently in patients who experienced MAb (Group 1) and who did not (Group 2); Table S4: Day of recovery (evaluated as independent variable), relates differently in patients who experienced MAb (Group 1) and who did not (Group 2); Figure S1: Examples of LUS in patient who recovered (upper panels) and who did not (lower panels). Stars indicated ultrasonographic image of B-lines.

Author Contributions: Conceptualization, S.C. and A.G.S.; methodology, S.C. and F.P.; validation, C.M., A.G.S. and G.L.; formal analysis, S.C.; investigation, S.C., M.S.M., C.A.P., E.S., A.F., F.A., F.S., A.G.S., F.P.; data curation, S.C. and M.S.M.; writing—original draft preparation, S.C., M.S.M. and A.G.S.; writing—review and editing, D.F.B., L.D., A.S., R.R. and A.V.; supervision, A.V. and R.R.; All authors have read and agreed to the published version of the manuscript.

Funding: This research received no external funding.

Institutional Review Board Statement: The study was conducted in accordance with the Declaration of Helsinki and approved by the Ethics Committee of University of Bari Medical School (protocol code n° 6357/2020).

Informed Consent Statement: Informed consent was obtained from all subjects involved in the study.

Data Availability Statement: The data are not publicly available due to ethical restriction.

Acknowledgments: This study was part of the training program for ultrasonographer of the Italian Society of Ultrasound in Medicine and Biology held by Stefania Longo in Internal Medicine "G. Baccelli"—AUOC Policlinico di Bari.

Conflicts of Interest: The authors declare no conflict of interest.

References

1. Cates, J.; Lucero-Obusan, C.; Dahl, R.M.; Schirmer, P.; Garg, S.; Oda, G.; Hall, A.J.; Langley, G.; Havers, F.P.; Holodniy, M.; et al. Risk for In-Hospital Complications Associated with COVID-19 and Influenza—Veterans Health Administration, United States, October 1, 2018–May 31, 2020. *MMWR Morb. Mortal. Wkly. Rep.* **2020**, *69*, 1528–1534. [CrossRef] [PubMed]
2. Chidambaram, V.; Tun, N.L.; Haque, W.Z.; Gilbert Majella, M.; Kumar Sivakumar, R.; Kumar, A.; Hsu, A.T.W.; Ishak, I.A.; Nur, A.A.; Ayeh, S.K.; et al. Factors associated with disease severity and mortality among patients with COVID-19: A systematic review and meta-analysis. *PLoS ONE* **2020**, *15*, e0241541. [CrossRef] [PubMed]
3. Berlin, D.A.; Gulick, R.M.; Martinez, F.J. Severe Covid-19. *N. Engl. J. Med.* **2020**, *383*, 2451–2460. [CrossRef] [PubMed]
4. Dougan, M.; Nirula, A.; Azizad, M.; Mocherla, B.; Gottlieb, R.L.; Chen, P.; Hebert, C.; Perry, R.; Boscia, J.; Heller, B.; et al. Bamlanivimab plus Etesevimab in Mild or Moderate Covid-19. *N. Engl. J. Med.* **2021**, *385*, 1382–1392. [CrossRef] [PubMed]
5. Seibel, A.; Heinz, W.; Greim, C.; Weber, S. Lungensonographie bei COVID-19. *Wien. Klin. Mag.* **2021**, *24*, 164–172. [CrossRef]
6. Cicco, S.; Vacca, A.; Cariddi, C.; Carella, R.; Altamura, G.; Solimando, A.G.; Lauletta, G.; Pappagallo, F.; Cirulli, A.; Stragapede, A.; et al. Imaging Evaluation of Pulmonary and Non-Ischaemic Cardiovascular Manifestations of COVID-19. *Diagnostics* **2021**, *11*, 1271. [CrossRef]
7. Bavaro, D.; Diella, L.; Solimando, A.; Cicco, S.; Buonamico, E.; Stasi, C.; Ciannarella, M.; Marrone, M.; Carpagnano, F.; Resta, O.; et al. Bamlanivimab and Etesevimab administered in an outpatient setting for SARS-CoV-2 infection. *Pathog. Glob. Health* **2022**, *116*, 297–304. [CrossRef]
8. Elsaghir, H.; Adnan, G. Best practices for administering monoclonal antibody therapy for coronavirus (COVID-19). In *StatPearls*; StatPearls Publishing: Tampa, FL, USA, 2022.
9. Gottlieb, R.L.; Nirula, A.; Chen, P.; Boscia, J.; Heller, B.; Morris, J.; Huhn, G.; Cardona, J.; Mocherla, B.; Stosor, V.; et al. Effect of Bamlanivimab as monotherapy or in combination with Etesevimab on viral load in patients with mild to moderate COVID-19: A randomized clinical trial. *JAMA J. Am. Med. Assoc.* **2021**, *325*, 632–644. [CrossRef]
10. Agenzia Italiana del Farmaco. *Definizione delle Modalita' e delle Condizioni di Impiego Dell'anticorpo Monoclonale Bamlanivimab-Etesevimab. (Determina n. DG/318/2021)*; Gazzetta Ufficiale: Rome, Italy, 2021; No. 66.
11. Xue, H.; Li, C.; Cui, L.; Tian, C.; Li, S.; Wang, Z.; Liu, C.; Ge, Q. M-BLUE protocol for coronavirus disease-19 (COVID-19) patients: Interobserver variability and correlation with disease severity. *Clin. Radiol.* **2021**, *76*, 379–383. [CrossRef]
12. Solimando, A.G.; Susca, N.; Borrelli, P.; Prete, M.; Lauletta, G.; Pappagallo, F.; Buono, R.; Inglese, G.; Forina, B.M.; Bochicchio, D.; et al. Short-Term Variations in Neutrophil-to-Lymphocyte and Urea-to-Creatinine Ratios Anticipate Intensive Care Unit Admission of COVID-19 Patients in the Emergency Department. *Front. Med.* **2021**, *7*, 625176. [CrossRef]
13. Carpenter, C.R.; Mudd, P.A.; West, C.P.; Wilber, E.; Wilber, S.T. Diagnosing COVID-19 in the Emergency Department: A Scoping Review of Clinical Examinations, Laboratory Tests, Imaging Accuracy, and Biases. *Acad. Emerg. Med.* **2020**, *27*, 653–670. [CrossRef] [PubMed]
14. Xu, X.W.; Wu, X.X.; Jiang, X.G.; Xu, K.J.; Ying, L.J.; Ma, C.L.; Li, S.B.; Wang, H.Y.; Zhang, S.; Gao, H.N.; et al. Clinical findings in a group of patients infected with the 2019 novel coronavirus (SARS-Cov-2) outside of Wuhan, China: Retrospective case series. *BMJ* **2020**, *368*, m606. [CrossRef]
15. McCreary, E.K.; Pogue, J.M. COVID-19 Treatment: A Review of Early and Emerging Options. *Open Forum Infect. Dis.* **2020**. [CrossRef]
16. Ferré, E.M.N.; Schmitt, M.M.; Ochoa, S.; Rosen, L.B.; Shaw, E.R.; Burbelo, P.D.; Stoddard, J.L.; Rampertaap, S.; DiMaggio, T.; Bergerson, J.R.E.; et al. SARS-CoV-2 Spike Protein-Directed Monoclonal Antibodies May Ameliorate COVID-19 Complications in APECED Patients. *Front. Immunol.* **2021**, *12*, 720205. [CrossRef] [PubMed]
17. Shi, R.; Shan, C.; Duan, X.; Chen, Z.; Liu, P.; Song, J.; Song, T.; Bi, X.; Han, C.; Wu, L.; et al. A human neutralizing antibody targets the receptor-binding site of SARS-CoV-2. *Nature* **2020**, *584*, 120–124. [CrossRef] [PubMed]
18. Cicco, S.; Mozzini, C.; Marozzi, M.; De Fazio, G.; Carella, R.; Vacca, A.; Cariddi, C.; Pappagallo, F.; Solimando, A.G.; Ria, R. Cardiovascular risk score may be useful in stratify death risk in hospitalized covid19 patients. *J. Hypertens.* **2022**, *40*, e172. [CrossRef]

19. Guzik, T.J.; Mohiddin, S.A.; Dimarco, A.; Patel, V.; Savvatis, K.; Marelli-Berg, F.M.; Madhur, M.S.; Tomaszewski, M.; Maffia, P.; D'Acquisto, F.; et al. COVID-19 and the cardiovascular system: Implications for risk assessment, diagnosis, and treatment options. *Cardiovasc. Res.* **2020**, *116*, 1666–1687. [CrossRef] [PubMed]
20. Başaran, S.; Şimşek-Yavuz, S.; Meşe, S.; Çağatay, A.; Medetalibeyoğlu, A.; Öncül, O.; Özsüt, H.; Ağaçfidan, A.; Gül, A.; Eraksoy, H. The effect of tocilizumab, anakinra and prednisolone on antibody response to SARS-CoV-2 in patients with COVID-19: A prospective cohort study with multivariate analysis of factors affecting the antibody response. *Int. J. Infect. Dis.* **2021**, *105*, 756–762. [CrossRef]
21. Masci, G.M.; Iafrate, F.; Ciccarelli, F.; Pambianchi, G.; Panebianco, V.; Pasculli, P.; Ciardi, M.R.; Mastroianni, C.M.; Ricci, P.; Catalano, C.; et al. Tocilizumab effects in COVID-19 pneumonia: Role of CT texture analysis in quantitative assessment of response to therapy. *Radiol. Medica* **2021**, *126*, 1170–1180. [CrossRef]
22. Sava, M.; Sommer, G.; Daikeler, T.; Woischnig, A.K.; Martinez, A.E.; Leuzinger, K.; Hirsch, H.; Erlanger, T.; Wiencierz, A.; Bassetti, S.; et al. Ninety-day outcome of patients with severe COVID-19 treated with tocilizumab—A single centre cohort study. *Swiss Med. Wkly.* **2021**, *151*, w20550. [CrossRef]
23. Guigon, A.; Faure, E.; Lemaire, C.; Chopin, M.C.; Tinez, C.; Assaf, A.; Lazrek, M.; Hober, D.; Bocket, L.; Engelmann, I.; et al. Emergence of Q493R mutation in SARS-CoV-2 spike protein during Bamlanivimab/Etesevimab treatment and resistance to viral clearance. *J. Infect.* **2022**, *84*, 248–288. [CrossRef] [PubMed]
24. Chang, M.C.; Lee, W.; Hur, J.; Park, D. Chest Computed Tomography Findings in Asymptomatic Patients with COVID-19. *Respiration* **2020**, *99*, 748–754. [CrossRef] [PubMed]
25. Inui, S.; Fujikawa, A.; Jitsu, M.; Kunishima, N.; Watanabe, S.; Suzuki, Y.; Umeda, S.; Uwabe, Y. Chest ct findings in cases from the cruise ship diamond princess with coronavirus disease (Covid-19). *Radiol. Cardiothorac. Imaging* **2020**, *2*, e200110. [CrossRef]
26. So, M.; Kabata, H.; Fukunaga, K.; Takagi, H.; Kuno, T. Radiological and functional lung sequelae of COVID-19: A systematic review and meta-analysis. *BMC Pulm. Med.* **2021**, *21*, 97. [CrossRef] [PubMed]
27. Watanabe, A.; So, M.; Iwagami, M.; Fukunaga, K.; Takagi, H.; Kabata, H.; Kuno, T. One-year follow-up CT findings in COVID-19 patients: A systematic review and meta-analysis. *Respirology* **2022**, *27*, 605–616. [CrossRef]
28. Munker, D.; Veit, T.; Barton, J.; Mertsch, P.; Mümmler, C.; Osterman, A.; Khatamzas, E.; Barnikel, M.; Hellmuth, J.C.; Münchhoff, M.; et al. Pulmonary function impairment of asymptomatic and persistently symptomatic patients 4 months after COVID-19 according to disease severity. *Infection* **2022**, *50*, 157–168. [CrossRef]
29. Smith, M.J.; Hayward, S.A.; Innes, S.M.; Miller, A.S.C. Point-of-care lung ultrasound in patients with COVID-19—A narrative review. *Anaesthesia* **2020**, *75*, 1096–1104. [CrossRef]
30. Cicco, S.; Cicco, G.; Racanelli, V.; Vacca, A. Neutrophil Extracellular Traps (NETs) and Damage-Associated Molecular Patterns (DAMPs): Two Potential Targets for COVID-19 Treatment. *Mediat. Inflamm.* **2020**, *2020*, 7527953. [CrossRef]
31. Cicco, S.; Vacca, A.; Cittadini, A.; Marra, A.M. Long-Term Follow-Up May be Useful in Coronavirus Disease 2019 Survivors to Prevent Chronic Complications. *Infect. Chemother.* **2020**, *52*, 407. [CrossRef]
32. Saltiel, A.R.; Olefsky, J.M. Inflammatory mechanisms linking obesity and metabolic disease. *J. Clin. Investig.* **2017**, *127*, 1–4. [CrossRef]
33. Monteiro, R.; Azevedo, I. Chronic inflammation in obesity and the metabolic syndrome. *Mediat. Inflamm.* **2010**, *2010*, 289645. [CrossRef] [PubMed]
34. Rocha, V.Z.; Libby, P. Obesity, inflammation, and atherosclerosis. *Nat. Rev. Cardiol.* **2009**, *6*, 399–409. [CrossRef] [PubMed]
35. Finelli, C. Obesity, COVID-19 and immunotherapy: The complex relationship! *Immunotherapy* **2020**, *12*, 1105–1109. [CrossRef]
36. Chen, P.; Nirula, A.; Heller, B.; Gottlieb, R.L.; Boscia, J.; Morris, J.; Huhn, G.; Cardona, J.; Mocherla, B.; Stosor, V.; et al. SARS-CoV-2 Neutralizing Antibody LY-CoV555 in Outpatients with Covid-19. *N. Engl. J. Med.* **2021**, *384*, 229–237. [CrossRef] [PubMed]

Disclaimer/Publisher's Note: The statements, opinions and data contained in all publications are solely those of the individual author(s) and contributor(s) and not of MDPI and/or the editor(s). MDPI and/or the editor(s) disclaim responsibility for any injury to people or property resulting from any ideas, methods, instructions or products referred to in the content.

Article

Patients with Diabetes Experienced More Serious and Protracted Sickness from the COVID-19 Infection: A Prospective Study

Muiez Bashir [1], Wani Inzamam [1], Irfan Robbani [1], Tanveer Rasool Banday [2,*], Fahad A. Al-Misned [3], Hamed A. El-Serehy [3] and Carmen Vladulescu [4]

1. Department of Radiodiagnosis and Imaging, SKIMS Soura, Srinagar 190011, India
2. Department of Anaesthesia, SKIMS Soura, Srinagar 190011, India
3. Department of Zoology, College of Science, King Saud University, Riyadh 11451, Saudi Arabia
4. Department of Biology and Environmental Engineering, University of Craiova, 200585 Craiova, Romania
* Correspondence: tanveerbanday91@gmail.com

Abstract: *Background and Objectives*: In December 2019, a flu-like illness began in the Chinese city of Wuhan. This sickness mainly affected the lungs, ranging from a minor respiratory tract infection to a severe lung involvement that mimicked the symptoms of Severe Acute Respiratory Syndrome (SARS). The World Health Organization (WHO) labelled this sickness as a pandemic in March 2020, after it quickly spread throughout the world population. It became clear, as the illness progressed, that people with concomitant illnesses, particularly diabetes mellitus (DM) and other immunocompromised states, were outmatched by this illness. This study was aimed to evaluate the correlation between Computed Tomographic Severity Score (CTSS) and underlying diabetes mellitus in coronavirus disease (COVID)-19 patients. *Materials and Methods*: This was a hospital-based prospective study in which a total of 152 patients with reverse transcriptase polymerase chain reaction (RT-PCR) positive COVID status who underwent high-resolution computed tomography (HRCT) of the chest were evaluated and categorized into mild, moderate and severe cases based on the extent of lung parenchymal involvement. A total score from 0–25 was given, based on the magnitude of lung involvement. Statistical analysis was used to derive a correlation between DM and CTSS, if any. *Results*: From our study, it was proven that patients with underlying diabetic status had more severe involvement of the lung as compared to non-diabetics, and it was found to be statistically significant ($p = 0.024$). *Conclusions*: On analysis of what we found based on the study, it can be concluded that patients with underlying diabetic status had a more prolonged and severe illness in comparison to non-diabetics, with higher CTSS in diabetics than in non-diabetics.

Keywords: COVID-19; RT-qPCR; HRCT; diabetes mellitus; computed tomographic severity score; immunocompromised

1. Introduction

In the Chinese city of Wuhan, the first instance of coronavirus disease 2019 (COVID-19), which was brought on by the SARS-CoV-2 coronavirus, was discovered in December 2019. The outbreak started in the Huanan seafood and livestock market in Wuhan, in the province of Hubei, and it gave some evidence of an animal to human transfer through the trade in seafood and live livestock. The virus quickly spread throughout the Chinese city of Wuhan and others by January 2020 [1]. It subsequently spread to other nations and continents, and in March 2020, the WHO proclaimed it to be a pandemic. It has been determined that the pathogen is a brand-new enveloped RNA coronavirus [2]. Electron microscopy has shown that the coronavirus is a spherical virus with a diameter of approximately 125 nm. These virions feature surface-based projections that resemble clubs. The coronavirus got its name because of these spikes, which make them resemble a solar corona. In the past, coronaviruses were believed to have a small involvement in human respiratory infections that were mild and self-limiting. Every year, 15–30% of respiratory tract infections are caused by endemic coronavirus infections in the human population [3]. The factors affecting the disease severity and mortality were still mainly unknown because it was a new ailment. The intensity of the symptoms is thought to be affected by several factors, including underlying health issues, patients over 65 years of age, and delayed hospitalization. A severe coronavirus infection is thought to be more likely to occur in patients with underlying medical conditions such as diabetes or high blood pressure. These patients also have a higher chance of dying from COVID-19 and are likely to be more vulnerable [4]. Despite the fact that COVID-19 has been linked to the dysfunction of numerous important organs, including the kidneys, liver, heart, brain, and gastrointestinal system, SARS-CoV-2 primarily targets the lung, and lung failure is the leading cause of death in COVID-19 patients. The respiratory epithelium is infected with SARS-CoV-2, which results in severe cough, increased mucus production, breathlessness, tightness of the chest, and wheezing. Pneumonia, the development of Acute Respiratory Distress Dyndrome (ARDS), and respiratory failure necessitating mechanical ventilation are the hallmarks of severe COVID-19 [5]. The severity of COVID-19 disease is exacerbated by the presence of underlying comorbidities. Moreover, these patients have a higher risk of hospitalization and an increased need for ICU admissions and ventilators. While they typically have the worst prognosis, individuals with infirmities should take all essential steps to prevent contracting SARS-CoV-2. These safety measures include avoiding close contact with others and practicing social distancing, regularly washing hands with soap and water or using an alcohol-based hand sanitizer, donning a face mask in public settings and avoiding being out in public unless absolutely essential [6]. Approximately 537 million individuals throughout the world have diabetes mellitus (DM), according to statistics [7]. India has been dubbed the "Diabetes Capital of the World" due to the high incidence of DM. In the Southeast Asian area, it is anticipated that the prevalence of diabetes will rise to 11.3% among people between the ages of 20 and 79. About 77 million Indian individuals had diabetes overall as of 2019, and by 2030, it is projected that this figure will increase to 100 million [8]. Patients with a CTSS of >18 have a greater probability of dying, and this score is a reliable predictor of mortality. Using an ideal CTSS cutoff in the visual scoring of lung involvement, the likelihood of mortality for COVID-19 patients could be precisely predicted [9]. The identification and continual evaluation of COVID-19 rely heavily on HRCT. In patients with COVID-19 pneumonia, the imaging findings include ground-glass opacities and/or consolidations. It has been determined that respiratory failure brought on by diffuse alveolar injury is the main cause of death. The production of hyaline membrane and severe inflammatory exudates in intra-alveolar spaces are correlated with the ground glass opacities. It was also discovered that people who died had severity scores that were greater than people who only had mild to moderate sickness [10]. China has been acknowledged as having made progress in the outbreak's containment. The ability of China to effectively combat this disease is due to its robust economy, an abundance of economic resources, a strong government, efficient policy execution, and national cohesion. China took drastic measures to stop the spread of the disease by segregating suspected patients, keeping a tight eye on contacts, collecting data effectively, and developing diagnostic and treatment methods quickly and effectively. To contain the pandemic, enormous quarantine facilities were constructed and set aside [11].

This study aimed to establish an association between the severity of COVID-19 and DM.

2. Materials and Methods
2.1. Study Design

The study was a prospective one carried out in a tertiary care hospital, namely SKIMS Soura. IEC clearance was obtained. The IEC number of our study is IEC-SKIMS/2022-466.

2.2. Inclusion Criteria

All patients with RT-PCR proven COVID-19 status who had undergone HRCT chest scans.

2.3. Exclusion Criteria

Patients with severe motion artefacts precluding CTSS assessment and those who had undergone contrast study.

2.4. Data Collection

The investigation of choice for diagnosis of COVID-19 is RT-PCR. Patients who had been diagnosed with COVID were subjected to HRCT chest scans. HRCT scans were performed between the 5th and 10th day after the onset of symptoms. Using 64-slice multidetector CT (SOMATOM, Siemens Health liners, Erlangen, Germany), HRCT chest scans were obtained with patients in the supine position and breath-holding. The following parameters were used: tube voltage of 120 kV, tube current of 100–200 mAs, collimation of 1.5–2.5 mm, and slice thickness of 1–2 mm. The HRCT chest scans were analyzed using lung and mediastinal window reconstruction algorithms. The data from the HRCT lung studies of 152 patients performed between March and June 2021, during the second wave of COVID-19, were prospectively collected and inspected to determine the connection between diabetes and COVID-19 severity. An experienced radiologist scrutinized the data to determine the CTSS of the COVID-19 lung infection. A numerical CT score was computed based on the grade of lung parenchymal involvement (range: 0–5 for each lobe; total score range: 0–25). CT severity score (CTSS), when computed, helps to classify patients into mild (0–11/25), moderate (12–18/25), and severe (>18/25) (Table 1). The lung lobar involvement was set side by side between diabetic and non-diabetic patients based on CTSS.

Table 1. Tabular representation of grading of COVID-19 patients based on CTSS.

CLASS	CTSS (out of 25)
MILD	0–11
MODERATE	12–18
SEVERE	>18

2.5. Statistical Analysis

The categorical variables were presented in the form of numbers and percentages (%). On the other hand, the quantitative data with normal distribution were presented as the means ± SD, and the data with non-normal distribution as median with 25th and 75th percentiles (interquartile range). The data normality was checked by using the Kolmogorov–Smirnov test. For the cases in which the data were not normal, we used nonparametric tests. The following statistical tests were applied for the results: The comparisons of the variables that were quantitative and not normally distributed in nature were analyzed using the Kruskal–Wallis test, and variables that were quantitative and normally distributed in nature were analyzed using ANOVA. Univariate and multivariate logistic regression was used to identify significant risk factors for a moderate/severe CTSS (Table 2). Data entry was performed in Microsoft EXCEL spreadsheet, and the final analysis was conducted with the use of Statistical Package for Social Sciences (SPSS) software ver. 25.0 (IBM, Chicago, IL, USA). A p value of less than 0.05 was considered statistically significant.

Table 2. Univariate logistic regression to identify significant risk factors of moderate/severe CTSS.

Variable	Beta Coefficient	Standard Error	p Value	Odds Ratio	Odds Ratio Lower Bound (95%)	Odds Ratio Upper Bound (95%)
Gender						
Female				1.000		
Male	−0.040	0.339	0.905	0.960	0.494	1.866
Diabetics	0.973	0.397	0.014	2.645	1.214	5.761

3. Results

In our study, a total of 152 patients were enrolled. Out of these, 98 were males and 54 were females (approximately 65% males and 35% females, as depicted in Table 3).

Table 3. Distribution of demographic and baseline characteristics of study.

Demographic and Baseline Characteristics		
Age (Years)	Frequency	Percentage
≤20 years	01	0.66%
21–40 years	26	17.11%
41–60 years	86	56.58%
61–80 years	37	24.34%
>80 years	02	01.32%
Mean ± SD	52.9 ± 13.7	
Median (25th–75th percentile)	50 (45–61.25)	
Range	18–88	
Gender		
Female	54	35.53%
Male	98	64.47%
Diabetics	37	24.34%

A total of 37 patients were diabetics (24.34%). Of these 152 patients, just one was below 20 years of age, and most of the patients were in the age group from 41–60 years, with a mean age of 53 years. Furthermore, in our study, 25 patients (16%) were or had a history of being smokers with varying pack years. Approximately 28 patients (18%) were on antihypertensives, although their blood pressure was under control. As many as five patients had chronic kidney disease (3.2%). Additionally, 12 patients were on inhalers for COPD (7.8%). Four patients were undergoing treatment for hematological malignancies (2.6%). In this study, three patients (1.9%) had incidental detection of lung masses, and two patients (1.3%) had lung nodules.

Patients were labelled into mild (0–11), moderate (12–18), and severe (>18) categories based on the severity of lung involvement (Figure 1).

Multivariate logistic regression was carried out to identify significant risk factors for moderate/severe CTSS (Table 4).

Table 4. Multivariate logistic regression to identify significant risk factors for moderate/severe CTSS.

Variable	Beta Coefficient	Standard Error	p Value	Odds Ratio	Odds Ratio Lower Bound (95%)	Odds Ratio Upper Bound (95%)
Diabetics	0.886	0.425	0.037	2.426	1.054	5.584

Moderate and severe categories were classified into one category, and the association between DM and severe COVID-19 was calculated. Out of 152 patients with COVID-19, 77 (50.66%) had a mild score; 68 (44.74%) patients had a score of 12–18, which suggests moderate involvement, and the remaining 7 (4.61%) patients had a severe form of lung parenchymal involvement (Table 5).

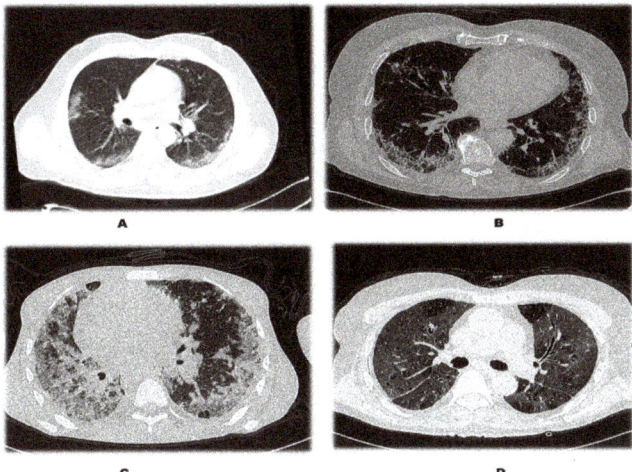

Figure 1. Pictorial representation of the severity of COVID-19 axial HRCT chest cuts with lung window demonstrating severity of disease: (**A**) Left upper—mild disease, (**B**) right upper—moderate disease, (**C,D**) severe disease.

Table 5. Association of CT severity score in patients with and without DM.

CT Severity Score	Patients without DM (n = 115)	Patients with DM (n = 37)	Total	p Value
0–11 {Mild}	65 (56.52%)	12 (32.43%)	77 (50.66%)	
12–18 {Moderate}	46 (40%)	22 (59.46%)	68 (44.74%)	0.024
>18 {Severe}	4 (3.48%)	3 (8.11%)	7 (4.61%)	
Total	115 (100%)	37 (100%)	152 (100%)	

Of the patients without diabetes, 65 (56.62%) were affected by a mild form of COVID-19, 46 (40%) had moderate disease, and four (3.48%) had a severe form of lung involvement as per CTSS scores (Table 5). Of patients with diabetes, 22 (59.46%) had a moderate and three (8.11%) had severe form of the disease (Figure 2). This relationship between COVID-19 infection and serious lung involvement was statistically significant (p = 0.024).

Additionally, it was found that lung involvement in COVID-19 was more severe in diabetics than in non-diabetics (as depicted in Table 5). Axial and coronal CT images of the patients depicted grading of COVID-19 infection (Figure 3).

Furthermore, it was found in our study that the mean duration of hospital stays of diabetics afflicted by COVID-19 was much higher than that of non-diabetics. We also noted longer recovery times for those COVID patients with underlying diabetes.

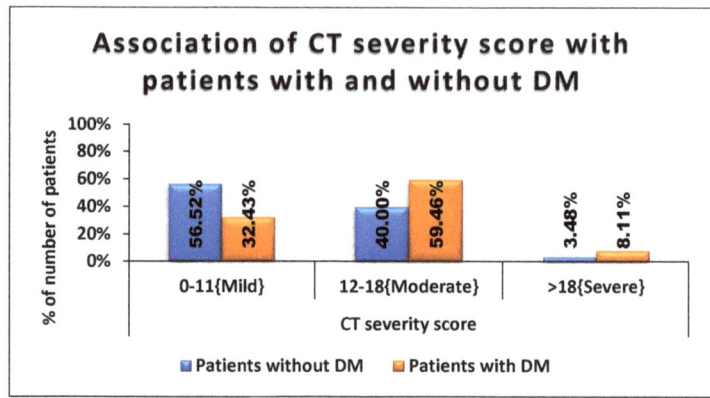

Figure 2. Association of CT severity score with patients with and without DM.

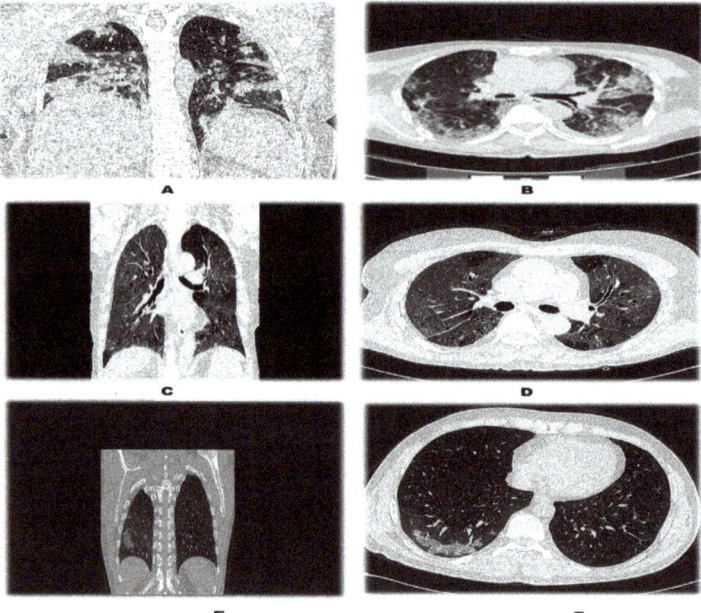

Figure 3. Axial and coronal cuts of patients with varying degrees of involvement of lung fields from severe to mild. (A,B) Coronal and axial cuts of a patient with severe involvement of the lung. (C,D) Coronal and axial cuts depicting moderate disease. (E,F) Mild involvement of lung field in a non-diabetic patient. The patient with severe lung involvement was the one who had underlying diabetes mellitus, clearly depicting severe involvement of lung fields.

4. Discussion

As per the data currently available, it is proven beyond doubt that underlying diabetic status significantly affects the clinical outcome of COVID-19 patients. Diabetics who contract COVID-19 have worse prognosis and a higher risk of death, although it has been found that symptomatology between diabetics and non-diabetics does not vary much in patients with COVID-19. Diabetes and other chronic diseases continue to present one of the biggest problems for healthcare professionals in terms of meeting patient's on-going needs. According to studies, preventing dysglycemia in diabetics can delay or even stop the development of their problems [12]. There is a high prevalence of diabetes in hospitalized COVID-19 patients. Moreover, underlying diabetes is a risk factor for higher mortality, especially in severely sick patients. Furthermore, it has been found that there is higher morbidity and mortality in diabetics who contract COVID-19 [13]. Diabetic patients with COVID-19 have a substantially higher mortality rate (15 vs. 2.3%) compared to COVID-19 patients without diabetes. Only a few research studies have demonstrated the link between diabetes and higher mortality risk (22–31% vs. 2–4%) [14]. The Computed Tomographic Severity Score (CTSS) is an indicator to gauge the severity of COVID-19 pneumonia [15]. Lower lobes of the lung, specifically the medial basal and lateral basal segments of the lung in both the right and left lower lobes, as well as the superior lingular segment, were the lobes most often afflicted [16].

Diabetic individuals showed a greater level of lung involvement than those without diabetes, which suggested a more serious lung infection, according to the quantifiable CT lung parenchymal involvement score [17]. A review of meta-analyses of various studies has shown that there is an association between COVID-19 and diabetic patients. The existence of chronic obstructive airway disease (COAD), acute kidney injury (AKI), underlying cardiac illness, advanced age, smoking and elevated BMI are additional variables that have been linked to poor outcomes in COVID-19 patients [18]. In a study conducted by the Chinese CDC, it was found that diabetics had a higher case fatality rate of 7.3%, in contrast to 2.3% in patients without diabetes. According to the Italian National Institutes of Health, 35.5% of patients who died from SARS-CoV-2 infection had diabetes [19]. Numerous other research studies have discovered that people with severe COVID-19 had a higher risk of developing diabetes, with some studies showing a two-fold increased risk. According to research by Wuhan Union Hospital using COVID-19 data, 21.2% of participants had diabetes, with radiographs showing advanced illness. Additionally, research from Italy similarly showed a 7.2% case fatality rate. Another study of ICU patients revealed that diabetes, hypertension, and cardiovascular disease were most frequently linked to serious illness [20].

There are clinically diagnosed stages of sickness in COVID-19 patients: the viremic stage, the acute stage, and the recovery stage. The joint action of the immune system's innate and adaptive mechanisms is responsible for this clinical result. Viral infections are recognized by the innate immune system through toll-like receptors (TLRs). The generation of type I interferons and NK cell defensive mechanisms then occurs. The production of antibodies by the adaptive immune system limits the persistence of infection. Lymphopenia observed during the acute stage of COVID-19 disease is caused by CD4+ and CD8+ apoptosis. The percentage of CD4+ and CD8+ T-cells in patients with COVID-19 was much lower than it was in the control group, according to the results of immunophenotyping [21]. The poor clinical outcomes in patients with diabetes and cardiovascular diseases afflicted with COVID-19 appear to be due to the down-regulation of the ACE2 protein. Human ACE2 is mostly expressed in the small intestine, adipose tissue, kidneys, lungs, and nasal epithelium. High levels of ACE2 expression in nasal mucosa are consistent with clinical findings indicating symptomatic COVID-19 patients have higher viral loads in their nasal cavities than in their throats, which may explain why some patients report losing their sense of smell. The ectodomain of ACE2 is a dissolvable protein that, despite maintaining its catalytic function, can be discovered in blood in the circulatory system [22]. Without a shadow of a doubt, people with hypertension or over the age of 60 have greater needs for both invasive and non-invasive ventilation [23].

Onder et al. observed that out of 355 patients who died due to COVID-19 in Italy, diabetic status accounted for the most common comorbidity (35.5%) attributed to COVID-19 death, followed by cardiac ischemic diseases (30%) [24]. Wang G. et al. found higher chances of diabetes in those with severe disease (10.8% vs. 5.4%) [25]. In Wuhan, Wang D. et al. noticed that patients who were in need of ICU treatment (n = 36) were more likely to have diabetes than patients who did not require ICU care (n = 102) (22.2% vs. 5.9%) [26].

In their study, Wu et al. noted an increased incidence of SARS in COVID-19 patients who had underlying diabetic status than in non-diabetics. Furthermore, it was found that among those who had developed SARS, those that were diabetic were more likely to experience death. It is unclear how diabetes worsens COVID-19, but multiple factors may play a role [27]. NK cells are a crucial type of effector in innate immunity. The function of these cells is crucial for adaptive immunity. These cells can also activate or suppress T-cell responses. Ineffective T cell, NK cell and complement action causes inadequate viral clearance and hence may play a role [28]. Adaptive and innate immunity are influenced by dysglycemia in diabetics, which might explain the increased incidence of viral and bacterial infections involving the lung in these patients [29]. COVID-19, beyond doubt, has been proven to be a pro-inflammatory state and thus might aggravate the cytokine storm. It is regarded as the root cause of ARDS and systemic dysfunction [30]. Adipokines have been discovered to play a significant role in how diabetics who also have COVID-19 fare [31]. Given this, it is important to note that in Type 2 diabetes, aberrant adipokine and cytokine production, and reduced immunity are all associated with an increased risk of infection [32]. Increased SARS-CoV-2 pathogenicity, which has been connected to diabetes, has been linked to higher plasminogen levels.

Diabetic patients are more likely to develop an aggressive form of coronavirus disease when their serum plasminogen levels are higher [33]. Serum levels of IL-6, ferritin, ESR, CRP, D-dimer and fibrinogen are significantly higher, as COVID-19 is an inflammatory and prothrombotic state [34]. An increase in ferritin, a protease enzyme associated with coronavirus entry into cells, may be the cause of increased viral replication in diabetes [35]. Patient care in diabetics should be improved to prevent morbidity issues and death [36]. For diabetics, self-care involves becoming aware of the complexity of their illness and acquiring the tools they need to manage it. Self-monitoring gives insight into one's current glycemic state, enabling therapeutic evaluation and directing changes to one's diet, exercise routine, and prescriptions in order to attain proper glycemic control [37]. Since the dysglycemia associated with diabetes is known to hinder patient recovery, diabetes and the COVID-19 condition may work in concert to adversely impair the patient's prognosis. It is possible that COVID-19 and diabetes have a reciprocal connection, with SARS-CoV-2 either aggravating existing diabetes or causing those who are not diabetic to develop it. SARS-CoV-2 penetrates cells via the ACE2 pathway, and as ACE2 is extensively expressed in the liver and pancreas, it may have a role in insulin resistance and decreased insulin production. The genesis and evolution of human diabetes are mostly dependent on beta-cell dysfunction because of the cumulative effects of hereditary and acquired factors [38].

There is no doubt that the pancreas of people with diabetes has a lower number of islet cells or a reduced number of beta cells. A crucial component of appropriate and proper beta-cell function is normal beta-cell integrity. Diabetes patients have been shown to have a beta-cell mass of less than 60%. Although beta-cell mass is known to be significant, Type 2 diabetes mellitus etiopathogenesis is more strongly associated with beta-cell number [39]. To reiterate, SARS-CoV-2 penetrates cells via the ACE2 pathway, and as ACE2 is extensively expressed in the liver and pancreas, it may have a role in insulin resistance and decreased insulin production [40]. Increased oxidative damage and inflammation caused by high blood sugar levels have been seen to alter the expression of genes linked to aberrant insulin production and an increase in apoptosis. Damage to mitochondria, cell proteins, nucleic acids, and lipids results from oxidative stress. Additionally, all of this results in endoscopic reticulum stress, which in Type 2 diabetes mellitus causes beta-cell death. Pancreatic beta-cell infection in susceptible people may eventually result in beta-cell autoimmunity [41]. After the COVID-19 outbreak has passed, we might witness a rise in the prevalence of autoimmune diabetes. Although we are well-versed in the immediate concerns of COVID-19 patients, its long-term effects also demand vigilance. The length of stay in the hospital was prolonged in diabetics patients as compared to non-diabetics [42].

Diabetic patients have longer hospital stays and a higher incidence of complications. Numerous studies have conclusively shown that diabetics do have longer hospital stays and greater admission rates (2–6 times higher than non-diabetics). Hospitalization rates and length of stay have been observed to be correlated with serum levels of HbA1c, insulin demand, duration of diabetes, and presence of complications, and the worse these factors, the worse will be the outcome of the patient [43]. Although the increasing problems in diabetes are still not fully understood, the immune system may contribute to the worsening of the condition. Since IL-6 can trigger an immune response and the formation of effector T cells, it is known to defend against infections [44]. The synthesis of acute phase reactants such as serum amyloid A, fibrinogen, C-reactive protein (CRP), haptoglobin, and alpha 1-antichymotrypsin is induced by IL-6, which is first produced in a local lesion during the early stages of inflammation [45]. It is also known that IL-6 alters the control of iron absorption and increases hepatic hepcidin synthesis. Additionally, it has been discovered that IL-6 increases VEGF synthesis, which promotes angiogenesis and increases vascular permeability [46].

Limitations

The limitations of our study were the limited sample size. In order to draw broader conclusions, further research including a larger sample size of individuals with complex clinical and laboratory correlations will be beneficial.

5. Conclusions

Our study has proven beyond doubt that diabetics are at escalated risk of developing a drastic form of COVID-19 illness. Any diabetic who has contracted COVID-19 should have strict glycemic control to avoid life-threatening complications thereof. Henceforth, diabetes is and should be considered one of the most important risk factors for developing a severe form of COVID-19 illness. Thus, the best way to reduce morbidity and mortality in diabetics is to avoid exposing them to COVID-19 positive patients.

Author Contributions: Conceptualization, M.B.; methodology, M.B., W.I. and I.R.; software, M.B.; validation, M.B., W.I. and I.R.; formal analysis, M.B., W.I., T.R.B., F.A.A.-M., H.A.E.-S., C.V. and I.R.; investigation, F.A.A.-M., H.A.E.-S., C.V. and M.B.; data curation, M.B., W.I., T.R.B. and I.R.; writing—original draft preparation, M.B., W.I., T.R.B. and I.R.; writing—review and editing. All authors have read and agreed to the published version of the manuscript.

Funding: This research received no external funding.

Institutional Review Board Statement: The study was conducted in accordance with the Declaration of Helsinki, and approved by the Institutional Review Board (or Ethics Committee) of SKIMS (IEC number of our study is IEC-SKIMS/2022-466) for studies involving humans.

Informed Consent Statement: Not applicable.

Acknowledgments: The authors would like to extend their sincere appreciation to the Researchers Supporting Project Number (RSP2023R24), King Saud University, Riyadh, Saudi Arabia. We sincerely appreciate Sheikh Mansoor Shafi Department of Human Genetics at SKIMS for proofreading the manuscript and for insightful advice and suggestions prior to publication.

Conflicts of Interest: The authors declare no conflict of interest.

References

1. Mohan, B.S.; Nambiar, V. COVID-19: An insight into SARS-CoV-2 pandemic originated at Wuhan City in Hubei Province of China. *J Infect. Dis. Epidemiol.* **2020**, *6*, 146. [CrossRef]
2. Hu, B.; Guo, H.; Zhou, P.; Shi, Z.L. Characteristics of SARS-CoV-2 and COVID-19. *Nat. Rev. Microbiol.* **2021**, *19*, 141–154. [CrossRef] [PubMed]
3. Fehr, A.R.; Perlman, S. Coronaviruses: An overview of their replication and pathogenesis. *Coronaviruses Methods Mol.* **2015**, *1282*, 1–23.
4. Chidambaram, V.; Tun, N.L.; Haque, W.Z.; Majella, M.G.; Sivakumar, R.K.; Kumar, A.; Hsu, A.T.; Ishak, I.A.; Nur, A.A.; Ayeh, S.K.; et al. Factors associated with disease severity and mortality among patients with COVID-19: A systematic review and meta-analysis. *PLoS ONE* **2020**, *15*, e0241541. [CrossRef]

5. Upadhya, S.; Rehman, J.; Malik, A.B.; Chen, S. Mechanisms of lung injury induced by SARS-CoV-2 infection. *Physiology* **2022**, *37*, 88–100. [CrossRef]
6. Sanyaolu, A.; Okorie, C.; Marinkovic, A.; Patidar, R.; Younis, K.; Desai, P.; Hosein, Z.; Padda, I.; Mangat, J.; Altaf, M. Comorbidity and its impact on patients with COVID-19. *SN Compr. Clin. Med.* **2020**, *2*, 1069–1076. [CrossRef]
7. Saeedi, P.; Petersohn, I.; Salpea, P.; Malanda, B.; Karuranga, S.; Unwin, N.; Colagiuri, S.; Guariguata, L.; Motala, A.A.; Ogurtsova, K.; et al. Global and regional diabetes prevalence estimates for 2019 and projections for 2030 and 2045: Results from the International Diabetes Federation Diabetes Atlas. *Diabetes Res. Clin. Pract.* **2019**, *157*, 107843. [CrossRef]
8. Paulsamy, P.; Ashraf, R.; Alshahrani, S.H.; Periannan, K.; Qureshi, A.A.; Venkatesan, K.; Manoharan, V.; Govindasamy, N.; Prabahar, K.; Arumugam, T.; et al. Social support, self-care behaviour and self-efficacy in patients with Type 2 diabetes during the COVID-19 pandemic: A cross-sectional study. *Healthcare* **2021**, *9*, 1607. [CrossRef]
9. Zakariaee, S.S.; Salmanipour, H.; Naderi, N.; Kazemi-Arpanahi, H.; Shanbehzadeh, M. Association of chest CT severity score with mortality of COVID-19 patients: A systematic review and meta-analysis. *Clin. Transl. Imaging* **2022**, *10*, 663–676. [CrossRef]
10. Lee, J.H.; Hong, H.; Kim, H.; Lee, C.H.; Goo, J.M.; Yoon, S.H. CT Examinations for COVID-19: A Systematic Review of Protocols, Radiation Dose, and Numbers Needed to Diagnose and Predict. *J. Korean Soc. Radiol.* **2021**, *82*, 1505–1523. [CrossRef]
11. Zhu, H.; Wei, L.; Niu, P. The novel coronavirus outbreak in Wuhan, China. *Glob. Health Res. Policy* **2020**, *5*, 6. [CrossRef]
12. Caballero, A.E.; Ceriello, A.; Misra, A.; Aschner, P.; McDonnell, M.E.; Hassanein, M.; Ji, L.; Mbanya, J.C.; Fonseca, V.A. COVID-19 in people living with diabetes: An international consensus. *J. Diabetes Its Complicat.* **2020**, *34*, 107671. [CrossRef]
13. Corona, G.; Pizzocaro, A.; Vena, W.; Rastrelli, G.; Semeraro, F.; Isidori, A.M.; Pivonello, R.; Salonia, A.; Sforza, A.; Maggi, M. Diabetes is most important cause for mortality in COVID-19 hospitalized patients: Systematic review and meta-analysis. *Rev. Endocr. Metab. Disord.* **2021**, *22*, 275–296. [CrossRef]
14. Yoo, S.J.; Goo, J.M.; Yoon, S.H. Role of Chest Radiographs and CT Scans and the Application of Artificial Intelligence in Coronavirus Disease 2019. *J. Korean Soc. Radiol.* **2020**, *81*, 1334–1347. [CrossRef]
15. Sayeed, S.; Faiz, B.Y.; Aslam, S.; Masood, L.; Saeed, R. CT Chest Severity Score for COVID 19 Pneumonia: A Quantitative Imaging Tool for Severity Assessment of Disease. *J. Coll. Physicians Surg. Pak.* **2021**, *31*, 388–392.
16. Rangankar, V.; Koganti, D.V.; Lamghare, P.; Prabhu, A.; Dhulipala, S.; Patil, P.; Yadav, P. Correlation between ct severity scoring and diabetes mellitus in patients with COVID-19 infection. *Cureus* **2021**, *13*, e20199. [CrossRef]
17. Dessie, Z.G.; Zewotir, T. Mortality-related risk factors of COVID-19: A systematic review and meta-analysis of 42 studies and 423,117 patients. *BMC Infect. Dis.* **2021**, *21*, 855. [CrossRef]
18. Ssentongo, P.; Zhang, Y.; Witmer, L.; Chinchilli, V.M.; Ba, D.M. Association of COVID-19 with diabetes: A systematic review and meta-analysis. *Sci. Rep.* **2022**, *12*, 20191. [CrossRef]
19. Yang, Y.; Zhong, W.; Tian, Y.; Xie, C.; Fu, X.; Zhou, H. The effect of diabetes on mortality of COVID-19: A protocol for systematic review and meta-analysis. *Medicine* **2020**, *99*, e20913. [CrossRef]
20. Angelidi, A.M.; Belanger, M.J.; Mantzoros, C.S. Commentary: COVID-19 and diabetes mellitus: What we know, how our patients should be treated now, and what should happen next. *Metab.-Clin. Exp.* **2020**, *107*, 154245. [CrossRef]
21. Fathi, N.; Rezaei, N. Lymphopenia in COVID-19: Therapeutic opportunities. *Cell Biol. Int.* **2020**, *44*, 1792–1797. [CrossRef] [PubMed]
22. Obukhov, A.G.; Stevens, B.R.; Prasad, R.; Li Calzi, S.; Boulton, M.E.; Raizada, M.K.; Oudit, G.Y.; Grant, M.B. SARS-CoV-2 infections and ACE2: Clinical outcomes linked with increased morbidity and mortality in individuals with diabetes. *Diabetes* **2020**, *69*, 1875–1886. [CrossRef]
23. Das, S.; Anu, K.R.; Birangal, S.R.; Nikam, A.N.; Pandey, A.; Mutalik, S.; Joseph, A. Role of comorbidities like diabetes on severe acute respiratory syndrome coronavirus-2: A review. *Life Sci.* **2020**, *258*, 118202. [CrossRef] [PubMed]
24. Abdi, A.; Jalilian, M.; Sarbarzeh, P.A.; Vlaisavljevic, Z. Diabetes and COVID-19: A systematic review on the current evidences. *Diabetes Res. Clin. Pract.* **2020**, *166*, 108347. [CrossRef] [PubMed]
25. Liu, Z.; Li, J.; Huang, J.; Guo, L.; Gao, R.; Luo, K.; Zeng, G.; Zhang, T.; Yi, M.; Huang, Y.; et al. Association between diabetes and COVID-19: A retrospective observational study with a large sample of 1,880 cases in Leishenshan Hospital, Wuhan. *Front. Endocrinol.* **2020**, *11*, 478. [CrossRef]
26. Landstra, C.P.; de Koning, E.J. COVID-19 and diabetes: Understanding the interrelationship and risks for a severe course. *Front. Endocrinol.* **2021**, *12*, 649525. [CrossRef]
27. Hussain, A.; Bhowmik, B.; do Vale Moreira, N.C. COVID-19 and diabetes: Knowledge in progress. *Diabetes Res. Clin. Pract.* **2020**, *162*, 108142. [CrossRef]
28. Paust, S.; Senman, B.; Von Andrian, U.H. Adaptive immune responses mediated by natural killer cells. *Immunol. Rev.* **2010**, *235*, 286–296. [CrossRef]
29. Chávez-Reyes, J.; Escárcega-González, C.E.; Chavira-Suárez, E.; León-Buitimea, A.; Vázquez-León, P.; Morones-Ramírez, J.R.; Villalón, C.M.; Quintanar-Stephano, A.; Marichal-Cancino, B.A. Susceptibility for some infectious diseases in patients with diabetes: The key role of glycemia. *Front. Public Health* **2021**, *9*, 559595. [CrossRef]
30. Ye, Q.; Wang, B.; Mao, J. The pathogenesis and treatment of the 'Cytokine Storm' in COVID-19. *J. Infect.* **2020**, *80*, 607–613. [CrossRef]
31. Jaganathan, R.; Ravindran, R.; Dhanasekaran, S. Emerging role of adipocytokines in type 2 diabetes as mediators of insulin resistance and cardiovascular disease. *Can. J. Diabetes* **2018**, *42*, 446–456.e1. [CrossRef]

32. Daryabor, G.; Atashzar, M.R.; Kabelitz, D.; Meri, S.; Kalantar, K. The effects of type 2 diabetes mellitus on organ metabolism and the immune system. *Front. Immunol.* **2020**, *11*, 1582. [CrossRef]
33. Gęca, T.; Wojtowicz, K.; Guzik, P.; Góra, T. Increased risk of COVID-19 in patients with diabetes mellitus—Current challenges in pathophysiology, treatment and prevention. *Int. J. Environ. Res. Public Health* **2022**, *19*, 6555. [CrossRef]
34. Elibol, E.; Baran, H. The relation between serum D-dimer, ferritin and vitamin D levels, and dysgeusia symptoms, in patients with coronavirus disease 2019. *J. Laryngol. Otol.* **2021**, *135*, 45–49. [CrossRef]
35. Xie, L.; Zhang, Z.; Wang, Q.; Chen, Y.; Lu, D.; Wu, W. COVID-19 and diabetes: A comprehensive review of angiotensin converting enzyme 2, mutual effects and pharmacotherapy. *Front. Endocrinol.* **2021**, *12*, 1541. [CrossRef]
36. Shrivastava, S.R.; Shrivastava, P.S.; Ramasamy, J. Role of self-care in management of diabetes mellitus. *J. Diabetes Metab. Disord.* **2013**, *12*, 1–5. [CrossRef]
37. Erener, S. Diabetes, infection risk and COVID-19. *Mol. Metab.* **2020**, *39*, 101044. [CrossRef]
38. Marchetti, P.; Bugliani, M.; Boggi, U.; Masini, M.; Marselli, L. The pancreatic β cells in human type 2 diabetes. *Diabetes Old Dis. New Insight* **2013**, *771*, 288–309.
39. Cerf, M.E. Beta cell dysfunction and insulin resistance. *Front. Endocrinol.* **2013**, *4*, 37. [CrossRef]
40. Ni, W.; Yang, X.; Yang, D.; Bao, J.; Li, R.; Xiao, Y.; Hou, C.; Wang, H.; Liu, J.; Yang, D.; et al. Role of angiotensin-converting enzyme 2 (ACE2) in COVID-19. *Crit. Care* **2020**, *24*, 422. [CrossRef]
41. Mine, K.; Nagafuchi, S.; Mori, H.; Takahashi, H.; Anzai, K. SARS-CoV-2 infection and pancreatic β cell failure. *Biology* **2022**, *11*, 22. [CrossRef] [PubMed]
42. Rathore, P.; Kumar, S.; Choudhary, N.; Sarma, R.; Singh, N.; Haokip, N.; Bhopale, S.; Pandit, A.; Ratre, B.K.; Bhatnagar, S. Concerns of health-care professionals managing COVID patients under institutional isolation during COVID-19 pandemic in India: A descriptive cross-sectional study. *Indian J. Palliat. Care* **2020**, *26* (Suppl. S1), S90. [PubMed]
43. Comino, E.J.; Harris, M.F.; Islam, M.F.; Tran, D.T.; Jalaludin, B.; Jorm, L.; Flack, J.; Haas, M. Impact of diabetes on hospital admission and length of stay among a general population aged 45 year or more: A record linkage study. *BMC Health Serv. Res.* **2015**, *15*, 12. [CrossRef]
44. Khalid, J.M.; Raluy-Callado, M.; Curtis, B.H.; Boye, K.S.; Maguire, A.; Reaney, M. Rates and risk of hospitalisation among patients with type 2 diabetes: Retrospective cohort study using the UK General Practice Research Database linked to English Hospital Episode Statistics. *Int. J. Clin. Pract.* **2014**, *68*, 40–48. [CrossRef] [PubMed]
45. Berbudi, A.; Rahmadika, N.; Tjahjadi, A.I.; Ruslami, R. Type 2 diabetes and its impact on the immune system. *Curr. Diabetes Rev.* **2020**, *16*, 442–449.
46. Tanaka, T.; Narazaki, M.; Kishimoto, T. IL-6 in inflammation, immunity, and disease. *Cold Spring Harb. Perspect. Biol.* **2014**, *6*, a016295. [CrossRef]

Disclaimer/Publisher's Note: The statements, opinions and data contained in all publications are solely those of the individual author(s) and contributor(s) and not of MDPI and/or the editor(s). MDPI and/or the editor(s) disclaim responsibility for any injury to people or property resulting from any ideas, methods, instructions or products referred to in the content.

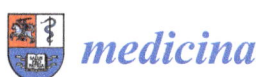

Case Report

Case Series of Patients with Coronavirus Disease 2019 Pneumonia Treated with Hydroxychloroquine

Tomohiro Tanaka [1,2], Masaki Okamoto [1,2,*], Norikazu Matsuo [1,2], Yoshiko Naitou-Nishida [1,2], Takashi Nouno [1,2], Takashi Kojima [1,2], Yuuya Nishii [1,2], Yoshihiro Uchiyashiki [1,2], Hiroaki Takeoka [1,2] and Yoji Nagasaki [3]

[1] Department of Respirology and Clinical Research Center, National Hospital Organization Kyushu Medical Center, 1-8-1 Jigyohama, Chuo-ku, Fukuoka 810-0065, Japan
[2] Division of Respirology, Neurology and Rheumatology, Department of Internal Medicine, Kurume University School of Medicine, 67 Asahi-machi, Kurume, Fukuoka 830-0011, Japan
[3] Department of Infectious Disease, National Hospital Organization Kyushu Medical Center, 1-8-1 Jigyohama, Chuo-ku, Fukuoka 810-0065, Japan
* Correspondence: okamoto_masaki@med.kurume-u.ac.jp; Tel.: +81-92-852-0700

Abstract: The efficacy of hydroxychloroquine (HCQ) therapy, a previous candidate drug for coronavirus disease 2019 (COVID-19), was denied in the global guideline. The risk of severe cardiac events associated with HCQ was inconsistent in previous reports. In the present case series, we show the tolerability of HCQ therapy in patients treated in our hospital, and discuss the advantages and disadvantages of HCQ therapy for patients with COVID-19. A representative case was a 66-year-old woman who had become infected with severe acute respiratory syndrome coronavirus 2 and was diagnosed as having COVID-19 pneumonia via polymerase chain reaction. She was refractory to treatment with levofloxacin, lopinavir, and ritonavir, while her condition improved after beginning HCQ therapy without severe side effects. We show the tolerability of HCQ therapy for 27 patients treated in our hospital. In total, 21 adverse events occurred in 20 (74%) patients, namely, diarrhea in 11 (41%) patients, and elevated levels of both aspartate aminotransferase and alanine transaminase in 10 (37%) patients. All seven grade ≥ 4 adverse events were associated with the deterioration in COVID-19 status. No patients discontinued HCQ treatment because of HCQ-related adverse events. Two patients (7%) died of COVID-19 pneumonia. In conclusion, HCQ therapy that had been performed for COVID-19 was well-tolerated in our case series.

Keywords: coronavirus disease 2019; hydroxychloroquine; severe acute respiratory syndrome

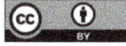

1. Introduction

The novel pathogen severe acute respiratory syndrome coronavirus 2 (SARS-CoV-2) caused an outbreak of viral pneumonia that became known as coronavirus disease 2019 (COVID-19), and was first reported in Wuhan, China in December 2019 [1]. After the initial outbreak, the illness rapidly spread globally [1].

The clinical studies of several drug candidates for COVID-19 therapy were globally performed [2,3]. However, the only drugs with evidence supporting reduced mortality against COVID-19 are corticosteroids. The RECOVERY trial, a controlled, open-label trial, suggested that 28-day mortality was lower in patients with moderate or severe COVID-19 who had received dexamethasone compared with those who had received standard care alone [4]. However, no benefit was seen in patients with mild COVID-19 [4]. In a prospective meta-analysis of 10,930 patients with COVID-19, compared with standard care or placebo, the administration of tocilizumab and interleukin-6 antagonists was associated with lower 28-day all-cause mortality [5].

Hydroxychloroquine (HCQ) and the 15-member macrolide antibiotic azithromycin (AZM) have been used for COVID-19 treatment, but were denied in therapeutic guidelines [6–12]. HCQ and chloroquine phosphate, which are widely used antimalarial drugs that are also used to treat autoimmune diseases such as systemic lupus erythematosus, exert antiviral effects by increasing the endosomal pH to a level exceeding that required for viral/cell fusion [13]. These drugs also interfere with the glycosylation of cellular receptors for SARS-CoV-2 [6–9,13]. Because macrolides prevent the production of proinflammatory mediators, cytokines, and reactive oxygen species both in vitro and in vivo [14], and control the exacerbation of underlying respiratory diseases such as asthma, panbronchiolitis, acute respiratory distress syndrome, and chronic fibrosing interstitial pneumonia [15–17], a combination therapy with HCQ and AZM has been used to treat COVID-19. SARS-CoV-2 real-time polymerase chain reaction-negative conversion rates in patients with COVID-19 after combined treatment with HCQ and AZM were 83% and 93% on disease Days 7 and 8, respectively [9]. However, a randomized, controlled, open-label platform (RECOVERY) trial compared the 28-day-mortality rates of 1561 patients who had received hydroxychloroquine and 3155 patients who had received standard care; the rate did not differ between the groups [10]. Additionally, retrospective cohort studies revealed that treatment with HCQ and/or AZM was not associated with significant differences in the incidence of intubation or death or the rate of inhospital mortality [11,12]. A recent WHO guideline recommended against administering HCQ for treatment of COVID-19 patients [18]. Moreover, there are concerns that HCQ may cause cardiovascular events, such as arrhythmia or cardiac arrest, in patients with COVID-19. Chorin et al. observed that, among 80 hospitalized SARS-CoV-2-infected patients who had received HCQ plus AZM, 30% exhibited corrected QT interval (QTc) prolongation of >40 ms, and 11% exhibited QTc prolongation of >500 ms [19]. The increase in the risk in cardiac arrest by HCQ and/or AZM is caused from drug-induced QT-interval prolongation and torsades de pointes (a form of polymorphic ventricular tachycardia) [19,20]. A retrospective study performed in New York suggested that the incidence of cardiac arrest was significantly higher in patients receiving both HCQ and AZM (15.5%), but not in those receiving HCQ (13.7%) or AZM (6.2%) alone, compared with patients who had received neither drug (6.8%) [12]. There were also no significant differences in the relative likelihood of abnormal electrocardiographic findings between the patient groups [12]. In the RECOVERY trial, patients who had received HCQ had a greater risk of death from cardiac causes (mean excess, 0.4%), although there was no difference in the incidence of new major cardiac arrhythmia compared with that in patients who had received standard care [10]. However, it is not yet clear whether treatment with HCQ and/or AZM increases the risk of cardiac events among Japanese patients with COVID-19.

In the present case series, we show the tolerability of HCQ therapy in patients treated in our hospital, and we discuss the advantages and disadvantages of HCQ therapy that had been performed for COVID-19 patients.

2. Case Report

2.1. Representative Patient

The clinical course and chest high-resolution computed tomography (HRCT) images of a representative case are shown in Figure 1. A 66-year-old woman visited her local hospital with intermittent shivering and a fever of >38 °C that improved without intervention in February 2020. Three days later, she visited our hospital in compliance with directions from the health center on the suspicion of a COVID-19 infection contracted from her husband, who had been diagnosed with COVID-19 pneumonia. The patient had no symptoms, and her chest radiographs were normal. However, patchy peripheral ground-glass opacities involving the subpleural area were visible in the lower-right lung lobe that were consistent with previously reported findings of COVID-19 pneumonia. She was admitted to our hospital and was diagnosed with COVID-19 pneumonia on the basis of positive results from a polymerase chain reaction (PCR) assay for SARS-CoV-2 from an oropharyngeal swab sample. Test results from similar samples for antigens of influenza, respiratory syncytial virus, and adenovirus were negative. The patient's medical history included only a mackerel allergy, and she had no history of smoking. Her vital signs on admission were as follows: respiratory rate, 18 breaths/min; oxygen saturation (SpO_2), 96% (room air); heart rate, 96 beats/min; blood pressure, 151/70 mmHg; and body temperature, 36.7 °C. Auscultation revealed no abnormal respiratory or heart sounds. Hematology and other laboratory examinations showed slightly elevated C-reactive protein (CRP; 0.62 mg/dL) and lactate dehydrogenase (LDH; 245 IU/mL) levels, with lymphocytopenia (610 cells/µL). The patient's clinical course and chest HRCT images are shown in Figure 1. At hospital admission, the patient was asymptomatic. However, on Day 4 after admission, she developed a fever (38.3 °C) and began treatment with levofloxacin (500 mg/day), lopinavir (800 mg/day), and ritonavir (200 mg/day). On Day 6, the lopinavir and ritonavir were discontinued because the patient developed diarrhea that was suspected to be an associated adverse effect. On Day 7, her condition deteriorated: her body temperature had increased to 39.1 °C, with elevated CRP (8.25 mg/dL) and LDH levels (353 IU/L), and decreased SpO$_2$ (91% on room air) compared with previous values. Therefore, we started treatment with hydroxychloroquine (400 mg/day). On Day 7, HRCT showed newly appeared ground-glass opacities in the right lung lobe. Interlobular septal thickening, perilobular opacities, and curvilinear lines were also observed in the peripheries of both lungs. After treatment with hydroxychloroquine, the patient's fever improved on Day 9, and all other symptoms improved on Day 15, as follows: CRP, 0.19 mg/dL; LDH, 208 IU/L; and SpO$_2$, 98% on room air. We confirmed that results from a PCR assay for SARS-CoV-2 were negative, and we stopped treatment with hydroxychloroquine. The patient was discharged on Day 16, and follow-up HRCT images obtained on Day 19 showed improvement in the lung changes. Her condition was stable after discharge. Grade 1 elevations in aspartate aminotransferase (AST) and alanine aminotransferase (ALT) levels, in accordance with the Common Terminology Criteria for Adverse Events version 5.0, both of which increased on Day 11 and normalized on Day 26, were suspected to be adverse effects of HCQ therapy.

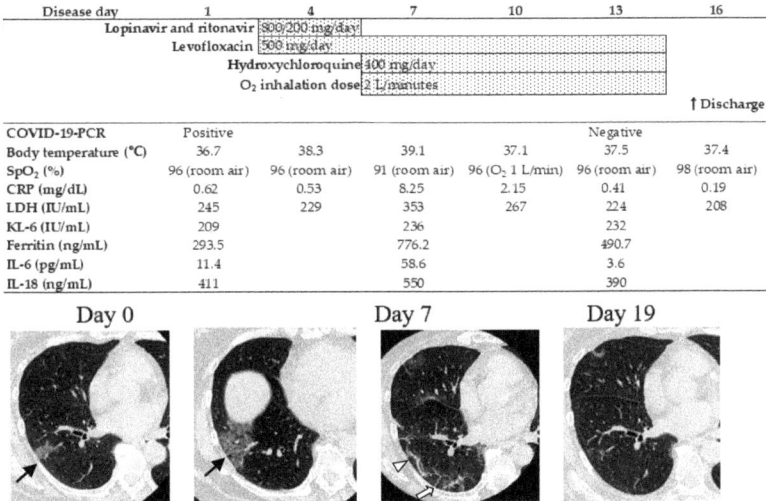

Figure 1. Clinical course of a representative case. O$_2$, oxygen; COVID-19, coronavirus disease 2019; PCR, polymerase chain reaction; SpO$_2$, oxygen saturation; CRP, C-reactive protein; LDH, lactate dehydrogenase; KL-6, Krebs von den Lungen-6, ground-glass opacitie; black arrow, interlobular septal thickening; white arrow, perilobular opacities and curvilinear line; arrow head.

2.2. Outcome of COVID-19 Patients Treated with HCQ

The patient characteristics, outcomes, and safety and tolerability of therapy in patients with COVID-19 who had received HCQ in our hospital in 2020 are shown in Tables 1 and 2. A total of 27 patients (23 males; median age, 56.0 years), including Cases 1 and 2, were diagnosed with COVID-19 pneumonia via SARS-CoV-2 PCR and were treated with HCQ.

COVID-19 severity in the 27 patients was mild in 6 (22%), moderate in 12 (44%), and severe in 9 (33%). Of the 27 patients, 18 (66%) received concurrent AZM, 8 (30%) received a concurrent corticosteroid, 3 (11%) received concurrent favipiravir, 2 (7%) received concurrent lopinavir and ritonavir, 2 (7%) received concurrent tocilizumab, and 1 (4%) received concurrent remdesivir. Of the patients, 21 required oxygen therapy, namely, mechanical ventilation for 4 patients, mask with a reservoir for 5, and nasal cannula for 12. The remaining 6 patients did not require oxygen therapy.

Table 1. Patient characteristics.

N	27	Pharmacological therapy	
Age (years)	56.0 (46.0–72.0)	HCQ alone	27 (100%)
Gender	23 (85%)	HCQ with AZM	18 (66%)
Smoker	12 (44%)	Favipiravir	3 (11%)
e: mild/moderate/severe	6 (22%)/12 (44%)/9 (33%)	Lopinavir and ritonavir	2 (7%)
Data at admission		Remdesivir	1 (4%)
Count of blood cells		Corticosteroid	8 (30%)
White blood cells (/uL)	4500.0 (3600.0–6000.0)	Tocilizumab	2 (7%)
Neutrophils (%)	73.2 (65.6–76.8)	Oxygen therapy	
Lymphocytes (%)	16.9 (14.0–25.2)	Nasal cannula	12
Platelets ($\times 10^4$/uL)	17.8 (14.1–21.4)	Oxygen mask with reservoir	6
Laboratory data		Mechanical ventilation	3
CRP (mg/dL)	4.6 (1.4–9.3)		
Lactate dehydrogenase (IU/L)	320.0 (234.0–471.0)		
Ferritin (ng/mL)	781.1 (371.8–1222.7)		
Interleukin-6 (pg/mL)	16.9 (11.6–58.3)		
D-dimmer (ug/mL)	0.90 (0.50–1.2)		

HCQ, hydroxychloroquine; AZM, azithromycin; SARS-CoV2, Severe acute respiratory syndrome coronavirus; PCR. polymerase chain reaction.

Table 2. Present and previous reports of HCQ therapy.

			Administration Dose (mg/day)		Duration of Administration (Days)		Main
	Design	N	HCQ	AZM	HCQ	AZM	Side Effect
Horby et al. [10] (RECOVERY trial)	RCT	4716	800 (loading dose) † 400 (maintenance dose)		6.0		Risk of death from cardiac causes
Geleris et al. [11]	Observational study	1376	600 (loading dose) 400 (maintenance dose)		5.0		N.D.
Rosenberg et al. [12]	Retrospective study	1438	400 in 90.3% of subjects	500 in 92.0% of subjects	N.D.	N.D.	Cardiac arrest in HCQ and AZM group
Gautret et al. [9]	Retrospective study	80	600	500 (loading dose) 250 (maintenance dose)	10.0	5.0	N.D.
The present study	Retrospective study	27	400	500 (p.o.) or 2000 mg (i.v.)	10.0 (6.0–12.0)	3.0 (3.0–3.5) (p.o.) 1.0 (i.v.)	Diarrhea

HCQ, hydroxychloroquine; AZM, azithromycin, RCT, randomized controlled trial; p.o., per oral; i.v., intravenous; N.D., no data. † 800 mg of HCQ were administered at 0 and 6 h followed by a maintenance dose of 400 mg every 12 h.

2.3. Tolerability of Treatment with HCQ in Patients with COVID-19

Table 2 shows the administration dose and duration of HCQ and AZM therapy in previous studies and the present study. In the present study, 400 mg of HCQ was administered to all patients, and the median duration of treatment was 10.0 (6.0–12.0) days. In 14 of the 18 patients treated with AZM, 500 mg was administered intravenously for 3.0 (3.0–3.5) days, and 4 patients received 2000 mg for 1 day. In a retrospective study in New

York, 908 (90.3%) of 1006 HCQ-treated patients received 400 mg of AZM [12]. Among 946 AZM-treated patients, 870 (92.0%) received a dose of 500 mg [12]. Similarly, AZM was administered orally to 454 (48.0%) patients and intravenously to 482 (50.9%) patients [12]. Although the administration period of HCQ was not stated, the median hospital stay was 7 days in both the HCQ + AZM and HCQ monotherapy groups in the study [12]. In a cohort study in France, HCQ was administered at a dose of 600 mg daily for 10 days combined with AZM at a dose of 500 mg on Day 1, followed by 250 mg daily for the next 4 days [9]. In a cohort study in New York City, HCQ was administered at a dose of 600 mg on Day 1 followed by 400 mg daily for a median of 5 days [11]. In the RECOVERY trial, 800 mg of HCQ was administered at 0 and 6 h followed by a maintenance dose of 400 mg every 12 h for a median of 6 days (interquartile range, 3–10 days) [10]. In our study, there was no significant difference in the cumulative dose and duration of treatment with HCQ and AZM compared with previous reports.

The details of the adverse events (AEs) that had occurred during HCQ treatment are presented in Table 3. We observed 47 AEs in 20 (74%) of 27 patients with COVID-19. The AE severities in accordance with the Common Terminology Criteria for Adverse Events version 5.0 were Grade 1 in 5 (19%) patients, Grade 2 in 8 (30%) patients, Grade 3 in 1 (4%) patient, Grade 4 in 5 (19%) patients, and Grade 5 in 2 (7%) patients. All Grade ≥ 4 AEs were associated with deterioration of COVID-19. Two patients eventually died of COVID-19, with the deaths occurring 44 days after the start of HCQ treatment in one patient, and 18 days after admission in the second patient. The most frequent AE was diarrhea, occurring in 11 of 27 (41%) patients. The most frequent AE in the blood laboratory tests was elevated AST and ALT levels, which occurred in 10 of 27 (37%) patients. Neither arrhythmia nor cardiac arrest was observed in any patient. Bacterial pneumonia occurred after beginning HCQ therapy in two patients who had been diagnosed with ventilation-associated pneumonia caused by methicillin-resistant *Staphylococcus aureus*. One of these patients developed sepsis, and methicillin-resistant *Staphylococcus aureus* was detected via blood culture. Of the 11 patients with diarrhea during hospitalization in the infectious disease ward, 9 (82%) recovered. The duration from the initial appearance of diarrhea to recovery was 1.0 (1.0–4.5) days. In the patients with AST and ALT elevation, the elevations resolved in 6 (60%) patients, and the durations from the appearance of AST and ALT elevation to recovery were 14.0 (9.0–35.0) and 9.5 (3.8–23.8) days, respectively. The discontinuation of HCQ was required in only two patients, both of whom died of deterioration of COVID-19. No patient discontinued HCQ treatment because of HCQ-related AEs. Furthermore, no patients required an HCQ dose reduction. Our data indicate no severe HCQ-related AEs that required the discontinuation of the drug.

Table 3. Adverse events experienced by patients.

		Recovering	Duration (days)		Grade of CTCAE ver. 5.0				
		Yes/No	From Start of HCQ to Appearance of AE	From Appearance to Improvement of AE	1	2	3	4	5
Number	27								
Incidence of more than 1 AEe	20 (74%)								
Highest severity of AE evaluated by CTCAE ver. 5.0-grade					5 (19%)	8 (30%)	1 (4%)	5 (19%)	2 (7%)
Discontinuation of HCQ Cause	Death of COVID-19 2								
Adverse event									
Diarrhea	11 (41%)	9/2	1.0 (1.0–4.0)	1.0 (1.0–4.5)	11	0	0	0	0
Appetite loss	1 (4%)	1/0	1.0	2.0	0	1	0	0	0
Cough	2 (7%)	1/1	4.5 (4.0–5.0)	3.0	2	0	0	0	0
Elevation of aspartate transaminase	10 (37%)	6/4	4.0 (3.0–8.8)	14.0 (9.0–35.0)	6	2	2	0	0
Elevation of alanine transaminase	10 (37%)	6/4	4.5 (3.0–9.5)	9.5 (3.8–23.8)	6	1	3	0	0
Elevation of creatinine	1 (4%)	1/0	13.0	38.0	0	0	1	0	0
Thrombocytopenia	1 (4%)	0/1	29.0		0	0	1	0	0
Bacterial pneumonia	2 (7%)	2/0	7.0 (3.0–11.0)	13.5 (9.0–18.0)	0	0	2	0	0
Sepsis	1 (4%)	0/1	42.0		0	0	1	0	0
Guillain–Barre syndrome	1 (4%)	1/0	14.0	11.0	0	1	0	0	0
Deterioration of COVID-19	7 (26%)	5/2	2.0 (1.0–8.0)	13.0 (5.5–15.0)	0	0	0	5	2

AE, adverse event; CTCAE, Common Terminology Criteria for Adverse Events; HCQ, hydroxychloroquine; COVID-19, coronavirus disease-2019.

3. Discussion

We reported a clinical case series of patients who had received HCQ for COVID-19. As the data in patients treated with HCQ therapy were not compared with those in the control group, it is not certain that the adverse events were caused in the present case series by COVID-19 or HCQ therapy. One of the most frequent AEs in the present study was diarrhea. This result is similar to the findings in previous studies of chloroquine or HCQ treatment that reported that gastrointestinal involvement, typically of mild severity, is one of the main AEs associated with this regimen [21,22]. Conversely, two clinical studies on COVID-19 reported diarrhea in only 4 of 80 (5%) patients and 85 of 735 (11.6%) patients who had been treated with HCQ [9,12]. Diarrhea may be caused by gastrointestinal tract infection in patients with COVID-19. A previous cohort study found that 2–10% of patients with COVID-19 presented with diarrhea, and SARS-CoV-2 RNA was detected in both stool and blood samples [23]. The second most frequent AE in this study was elevated AST and ALT levels. However, this was an uncommon finding in previous reports of HCQ therapy; thus, the main cause of transaminase elevation may not have been HCQ therapy [19,21]. Previous cohort studies of patients with COVID-19 in China indicated that the incidence of transaminase elevation ranged from 16.1% to 53.1% [1,24,25]. Transaminase elevation in patients with COVID-19 may be caused by direct liver injury by SARS-CoV-2 via angiotensin-converting enzyme-2 in cholangiocytes, cytokine storm, or pneumonia-associated hypoxia [24,25]. In the present study, all episodes of diarrhea and transaminase elevation were Grade 1–2 in severity, and none required HCQ discontinuation.

In contrast to previous studies on HCQ therapy for COVID-19, none of our patients exhibited arrhythmia or cardiac arrest after commencing HCQ and/or AZM therapy [12]. Electrocardiograms performed in a previous study of patients treated with HCQ for connective tissue disease revealed that the heart conditions of these patients, including QTc intervals, were not different from those of healthy controls [26]. The rate of heart conduction disorders was similar to that expected in the general population. The cause of the difference in the incidence of arrhythmia and cardiac arrest between previous studies and the present study is unknown. Twelve-lead electrocardiogram (ECG) examination on admission or ECG monitoring were not performed in all of the present case series. One of the study limitations is that diagnostic tools for detecting arrhythmia may differ from those of previous studies of HCQ and/or AZM therapy. An important risk factor for arrhythmia associated with HCQ exposure is QTc prolongation. The administration of certain drugs, such as H2 blockers and antipsychotics, can cause long QT syndrome (LQTS) [20]. Additionally, race-related differences in the prevalence of LQTS-related gene mutations could have influenced our study results. The compound mutations of LQTS-related genes were observed in 8.4% of 310 Japanese probands with genotyped LQTS [27]. Moreover, Itoh et al. reported that the gene mutation causing congenital LQTS was present in patients diagnosed with drug-induced LQTS [28]. We could not perform genetic testing in the present study. This limitation of the present study should be addressed in future research. The cumulative doses and durations of treatment with HCQ and AZM in the present study were not lower than those of previous observational studies and randomized controlled trials; therefore, it is unlikely that any differences affected drug tolerability [10,15–17]. The cause of the difference in the incidence of severe cardiac events between previous studies and the present study may be related to other factors, such as differences in the incidence of QT prolongation associated with race or concomitant drug therapy. The present case series supports the tolerability of HCQ therapy in Japanese patients with COVID-19. Recently, Samuel et al. discussed that HCQ may have potential as a therapeutic agent for long COVID-19 but not acute symptoms because HCQ can inhibit unremitting inflammatory response, MHC class II-mediated autoantigen presentation, a sustained endotheliopathy due to microthrombi shown in long COVID-19. However, more prospective trials are needed to prove the therapeutic efficacy of HCQ for long COVID-19 [29,30].

The present case series had some limitations. First, the present case series had a small population and were not compared with control subjects. Second, as mentioned above, the diagnostic tools for detecting arrhythmia were not unified. However, the preliminary results of tolerability of HCQ therapy for Japanese COVID-19 patients may contribute to the study of HCQ for other conditions such as long COVID-19.

4. Conclusions

In conclusion, treatment with HCQ for COVID-19 was well-tolerated in our case series.

Author Contributions: Conceptualization, T.T., M.O. and Y.N. (Yoji Nagasaki); methodology, T.T., M.O. and Y.N. (Yoji Nagasaki); validation, T.T., M.O., N.M., Y.N.-N., T.N., T.K., Y.N. (Yuuya Nishii), Y.U., H.T. and Y.N. (Yoji Nagasaki); formal analysis, T.T., M.O., N.M., Y.N.-N., T.N., T.K., Y.N. (Yuuya Nishii), Y.U., H.T. and Y.N. (Yoji Nagasaki); investigation, T.T., M.O., N.M., Y.N.-N., T.N., T.K., Y.N. (Yuuya Nishii), Y.U., H.T. and Y.N. (Yoji Nagasaki); resources, T.T., M.O., N.M., Y.N.-N., T.N., T.K., Y.N. (Yuuya Nishii), Y.U., H.T. and Y.N. (Yoji Nagasaki); data curation, T.T., M.O. and Y.N. (Yoji Nagasaki); writing—original draft preparation, T.T.; writing—review and editing, all authors; supervision, M.O. and Y.N. (Yoji Nagasaki); project administration, M.O. and Y.N. (Yoji Nagasaki); funding acquisition, M.O. All authors have read and agreed to the published version of the manuscript.

Funding: This research received no external funding.

Institutional Review Board Statement: The study was conducted in accordance with the guidelines of the Declaration of Helsinki and approved by the Institutional Review Board of the National Hospital Organization Kyushu Medical Center (approval number 20C059; 24 June 2020).

Informed Consent Statement: Informed consent was obtained in the form of an opt-out between the date of approval and 31 July 2021 for the analyses of biomarkers measured in clinical practice, and the measurement and analysis of noncommercialized biomarkers in residual serum.

Data Availability Statement: The data presented in this study are available on request from the corresponding author. The data are not publicly available due to ethical considerations.

Acknowledgments: We thank the nurse specialists and other medical staff of the infectious disease control team in the National Hospital Organization Kyushu Medical Center who participated in administering the therapy to the patients included in this study.

Conflicts of Interest: The authors declare no conflict of interest.

References

1. Huang, C.; Wang, Y.; Li, X.; Ren, L.; Zhao, J.; Hu, Y.; Zhang, L.; Fan, G.; Xu, J.; Gu, X.; et al. Clinical features of patients infected with 2019 novel coronavirus in Wuhan, China. *Lancet* **2020**, *395*, 497–506. [CrossRef]
2. Sharun, K.; Tiwari, R.; Yatoo, M.I.; Natesan, S.; Megawati, D.; Singh, K.P.; Michalak, I.; Dhama, K. A comprehensive review on pharmacologic agents, immunotherapies and supportive therapeutics for COVID-19. *Narra J.* **2020**, *2*, e92. [CrossRef]
3. Masyeni, S.; Iqhrammullah, M.; Frediansyah, A.; Nainu, F.; Tallei, T.; Emran, T.B.; Ophinni, Y.; Dhama, K.; Harapan, H. Molnupiravir: A lethal mutagenic drug against rapidly mutating severe acute respiratory syndrome coronavirus 2-A narrative review. *J. Med. Virol.* **2022**, *94*, 3006–3016. [CrossRef] [PubMed]
4. Recovery Collaborative Group; Horby, P.; Lim, W.S.; Emberson, J.R.; Mafham, M.; Bell, J.L.; Linsell, L.; Staplin, N.; Brightling, C.; Ustianowski, A.; et al. Dexamethasone in hospitalized patients with COVID-19. *N. Engl. J. Med.* **2021**, *384*, 693–704.
5. WHO Rapid Evidence Appraisal for COVID-19 Therapies (REACT) Working Group; Shankar-Hari, M.; Vale, C.L.; Godolphin, P.J.; Fisher, D.; Higgins, J.P.T.; Spiga, F.; Savovic, J.; Tierney, J.; Baron, G.; et al. Association between administration of IL-6 antagonists and mortality among patients hospitalized for COVID-19: A meta-analysis. *JAMA* **2021**, *326*, 499–518. [CrossRef]
6. Lamontagne, F.; Agarwal, A.; Rochwerg, B.; Siemieniuk, R.A.; Agoritsas, T.; Askie, L.; Lytvyn, L.; Leo, Y.S.; Macdonald, H.; Zeng, L.; et al. A living WHO guideline on drugs for COVID-19. *BMJ* **2020**, *370*, m3379. [CrossRef]
7. Gao, J.; Tian, Z.; Yang, X. Breakthrough: Chloroquine phosphate has shown apparent efficacy in treatment of COVID-19 associated pneumonia in clinical studies. *Biosci. Trends* **2020**, *14*, 72–73. [CrossRef]
8. Wang, M.; Cao, R.; Zhang, L.; Yang, X.; Liu, J.; Xu, M.; Zhengli Shi, Z.; Hu, Z.; Zhong, W.; Xiao, G. Remdesivir and chloroquine effectively inhibit the recently emerged novel coronavirus (2019-nCoV) in vitro. *Cell Res.* **2020**, *30*, 269–271. [CrossRef] [PubMed]
9. Gautret, P.; Lagier, J.C.; Parola, P.; Hoang, V.T.; Meddeb, L.; Sevestre, J.; Mailhe, M.; Doudier, B.; Aubry, C.; Amrane, S.; et al. Clinical and microbiological effect of a combination of hydroxychloroquine and azithromycin in 80 COVID-19 patients with at least a six-day follow up: A pilot observational study. *Travel Med. Infect. Dis.* **2020**, *34*, 101663. [CrossRef]
10. Recovery Collaborative Group; Horby, P.; Mafham, M.; Linsell, L.; Bell, J.L.; Staplin, N.; Emberson, J.R.; Wiselka, M.; Ustianowski, A.; Elmahi, E.; et al. Effect of hydroxychloroquine in hospitalized patients with COVID-19. *N. Engl. J. Med.* **2020**, *383*, 2030–2040. [PubMed]

11. Geleris, J.; Sun, Y.; Platt, J.; Zucker, J.; Baldwin, M.; Hripcsak, G.; Labella, A.; Manson, D.K.; Kubin, C.; Barr, R.G.; et al. Observational study of hydroxychloroquine in hospitalized patients with COVID-19. *N. Engl. J. Med.* **2020**, *382*, 2411–2418. [CrossRef]
12. Rosenberg, E.S.; Dufort, E.M.; Udo, T.; Wilberschied, L.A.; Kumar, J.; Tesoriero, J.; Weinberg, P.; Kirkwood, J.; Muse, A.; DeHovitz, J.; et al. Association of treatment with hydroxychloroquine or azithromycin with in-hospital mortality in patients with COVID-19 in New York state. *JAMA* **2020**, *323*, 2493–2502. [CrossRef] [PubMed]
13. Savarino, A.; Di Trani, L.; Donatelli, I.; Cauda, R.; Cassone, A. New insights into the antiviral effects of chloroquine. *Lancet Infect. Dis.* **2006**, *6*, 67–69. [CrossRef] [PubMed]
14. Kanoh, S.; Rubin, B.K. Mechanisms of action and clinical application of macrolides as immunomodulatory medications. *Clin. Microbiol. Rev.* **2010**, *23*, 590–615. [CrossRef]
15. Zarogoulidis, P.; Papanas, N.; Kioumis, I.; Chatzaki, E.; Maltezos, E.; Zarogoulidis, K. Macrolides: From in vitro anti-inflammatory and immunomodulatory properties to clinical practice in respiratory diseases. *Eur. J. Clin. Pharmacol.* **2012**, *68*, 479–503. [CrossRef]
16. Kawamura, K.; Ichikado, K.; Suga, M.; Yoshioka, M. Efficacy of azithromycin for treatment of acute exacerbation of chronic fibrosing interstitial pneumonia: A prospective, open-label study with historical controls. *Respiration* **2014**, *87*, 478–484. [CrossRef] [PubMed]
17. Walkey, A.J.; Wiener, R.S. Macrolide antibiotics and survival in patients with acute lung injury. *Chest* **2012**, *141*, 1153–1159. [CrossRef]
18. Therapeutics and COVID-19: Living Guideline. Available online: https://www.who.int/publications/i/item/WHO-2019-nCoV-therapeutics-2022.4 (accessed on 7 March 2023).
19. Chorin, E.; Dai, M.; Shulman, E.; Wadhwani, L.; Bar-Cohen, R.; Barbhaiya, C.; Aizer, A.; Holmes, D.; Bernstein, S.; Spinelli, M.; et al. The QT interval in patients with COVID-19 treated with hydroxychloroquine and azithromycin. *Nat. Med.* **2020**, *26*, 808–809. [CrossRef]
20. Beitland, S.; Platou, E.S.; Sunde, K. Drug-induced long QT syndrome and fatal arrhythmias in the intensive care unit. *Acta Anaesthesiol. Scand.* **2014**, *58*, 266–272. [CrossRef]
21. Morand, E.F.; McCloud, P.I.; Littlejohn, G.O. Continuation of long term treatment with hydroxychloroquine in systemic lupus erythematosus and rheumatoid arthritis. *Ann. Rheum. Dis.* **1992**, *51*, 1318–1321. [CrossRef]
22. Ruis-Irastorza, G.; Ramos-Casals, M.; Brito-Zeron, P.; Khamashta, M.A. Clinical efficacy and side effects of antimalarials in systemic lupus erythematosus: A systematic review. *Ann. Rheum. Dis.* **2010**, *69*, 20–28. [CrossRef] [PubMed]
23. Yeo, C.; Kaushal, S.; Yeo, D. Enteric involvement of coronaviruses: Is faecal-oral transmission of SARS-CoV-2 possible? *Lancet. Gastroenterol. Hepatol.* **2020**, *5*, 335–337. [CrossRef]
24. Singh, S.; Khan, A. Clinical characteristics and outcomes of coronavirus disease 2019 among patients with preexisting liver disease in the United States: A multicenter research network study. *Gastroenterology* **2020**, *159*, 768–771. [CrossRef]
25. Zhang, C.; Shi, L.; Wang, F.S. Liver injury in COVID-19: Management and challenges. *Lancet. Gastroenterol. Hepatol.* **2020**, *5*, 428–430. [CrossRef] [PubMed]
26. Costedoat-Chalumeau, N.; Hulot, J.S.; Amoura, Z.; Leroux, G.; Lechat, P.; Funck-Brentano, C.; Piette, J.C. Heart conduction disorders related to antimalarials toxicity: An analysis of electrocardiograms in 85 patients treated with hydroxychloroquine for connective tissue diseases. *Rheumatology* **2007**, *46*, 808–810. [CrossRef]
27. Itoh, H.; Shimizu, W.; Hayashi, K.; Yamagata, K.; Sakaguchi, T.; Ohno, S.; Makiyama, T.; Akao, M.; Ai, T.; Noda, T.; et al. Long QT syndrome with compound mutations is associated with a more severe phenotype: A Japanese multicenter study. *Heart Rhythm.* **2010**, *7*, 1411–1418. [CrossRef] [PubMed]
28. Itoh, H.; Sakaguchi, T.; Ding, W.G.; Watanabe, E.; Watanabe, I.; Nishio, Y.; Makiyama, T.; Ohno, S.; Akao, M.; Higashi, Y.; et al. Latent genetic backgrounds and molecular pathogenesis in drug-induced long-QT syndrome. *Circ. Arrhythm. Electrophysiol.* **2009**, *2*, 511–523. [CrossRef] [PubMed]
29. Fahriani, M.; Ilmawan, M.; Fajar, J.K.; Maliga, H.A.; Frediansyah, A.; Masyeni, S.; Yusuf, H.; Nainu, F.; Rosiello, F.; Sirinam, S.; et al. Persistence of long COVID symptoms in COVID-19 survivors worldwide and its potential pathogenesis—A systematic review and meta-analysis. *Narra J.* **2021**, *1*, e36. [CrossRef]
30. Samuel, S.Y.; Wang, S.S.Y.; Xu, C. Hydroxychloroquine: Is there a role in long COVID? *Clin. Rheumatol.* **2023**, *42*, 977–978.

Disclaimer/Publisher's Note: The statements, opinions and data contained in all publications are solely those of the individual author(s) and contributor(s) and not of MDPI and/or the editor(s). MDPI and/or the editor(s) disclaim responsibility for any injury to people or property resulting from any ideas, methods, instructions or products referred to in the content.

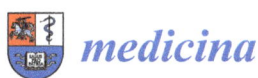

Article

Thoracic Mobilization and Respiratory Muscle Endurance Training Improve Diaphragm Thickness and Respiratory Function in Patients with a History of COVID-19

Yang-Jin Lee

Department of Physical Therapy, Gyeongbuk College, 77 Daehang-ro, Yeongju-si 36133, Gyeongsangbuk-do, Republic of Korea; ptyangjin2@naver.com; Tel.: +82-54-630-5265

Abstract: *Background and Objectives*: Common problems in people with COVID-19 include decreased respiratory strength and function. We investigated the effects of *thoracic mobilization and respiratory muscle endurance training* (TMRT) and lower limb ergometer (LE) training on diaphragm thickness and respiratory function in patients with a history of COVID-19. *Materials and Methods*: In total, 30 patients were randomly divided into a TMRT training group and an LE training group. The TMRT group performed thoracic mobilization and respiratory muscle endurance training for 30 min three times a week for 8 weeks. The LE group performed lower limb ergometer training for 30 min three times a week for 8 weeks. The participants' diaphragm thickness was measured via rehabilitative ultrasound image (RUSI) and a respiratory function test was conducted using a MicroQuark spirometer. These parameters were measured before the intervention and 8 weeks after the intervention. *Results*: There was a significant difference ($p < 0.05$) between the results obtained before and after training in both groups. Right diaphragm thickness at rest, diaphragm thickness during contraction, and respiratory function were significantly more improved in the TMRT group than in the LE group ($p < 0.05$). *Conclusions*: In this study, we confirmed the effects of TMRT training on diaphragm thickness and respiratory function in patients with a history of COVID-19.

Keywords: COVID-19; diaphragm; thoracic mobilization; respiratory function

Citation: Lee, Y.-J. Thoracic Mobilization and Respiratory Muscle Endurance Training Improve Diaphragm Thickness and Respiratory Function in Patients with a History of COVID-19. *Medicina* **2023**, *59*, 906. https://doi.org/10.3390/medicina59050906

Academic Editors: Masaki Okamoto and Patrick Geraghty

Received: 17 March 2023
Revised: 2 May 2023
Accepted: 3 May 2023
Published: 9 May 2023

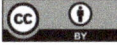

Copyright: © 2023 by the author. Licensee MDPI, Basel, Switzerland. This article is an open access article distributed under the terms and conditions of the Creative Commons Attribution (CC BY) license (https://creativecommons.org/licenses/by/4.0/).

1. Introduction

Common COVID-19 infection symptoms include cough, fever (37.5 °C or higher), fatigue, and shortness of breath, while other reported symptoms include weakness, malaria, respiratory distress, muscle pain, and sore throat. As such, the symptoms of COVID-19 patients range from asymptomatic to severe respiratory failure, and about 10% have severe dyspnea and abnormal findings of ground glass shadows in chest computed tomography [1–3].

In patients with respiratory problems, reduced respiratory efficiency and altered respiratory mechanisms should be corrected by maintaining adequate chest expansion, ventilation, and lung capacity [4].

Joint mobilization exercises of the spinal segments improve muscle efficiency by reducing the excessive use of and strengthening the erector spinae muscle; additionally, these exercises improve performance by allowing the use of appropriate muscles [5]. Moreover, improving the mobility of the muscles surrounding the joint can help optimize joint movement [6]. Watchie (2010) [7] reported that joint mobilization exercises for the thoracic region and backbone resolve ventilation inefficiency caused by pump dysfunction of the chest. Magee (2014) [8] suggested that the correction of chest cage deformations and exercises to improve chest wall flexibility should be performed to relieve the pressure on the lung parenchyma before irreversible damage to the pulmonary blood vessels occurs. Furthermore, Kim and Kim (2022) [9] observed significant differences in respiratory function and diaphragm muscle thickness after thoracic and lumbar stabilization exercises and upper extremity ergometer breathing training in 30 patients who had recovered from COVID-19 compared to the control group.

Respiratory exercise during hospitalization is a conservative treatment modality and is important for increasing respiratory muscle strength, coughing ability, chest wall mobility, and pulmonary ventilation [10]. Respiratory exercises include breathing using the diaphragm, which is the main inspiratory muscle, exhaling through pursed lips to reduce pain, and evoked spirometry to strengthen the inspiratory muscles [11]. Inspiratory muscle training (IMT) improves muscle strength and endurance by applying a load to the transverse and auxiliary inspiratory muscles [12]. IMT is an effective and safe method for improving respiratory function, cardiorespiratory capacity, activities of daily living, and quality of life; relieving dyspnea; and enhancing endurance in patients with brain injuries [13,14].

By comparing exhalation exercise, inhalation exercise, and interventional training that combines inhalation and exhalation, Tout (2013) [15] showed that IMT helps improve pulmonary function. Moodie et al. (2011) [12] reported that applying a load to the diaphragm and synergistic inspiratory muscles helps improve muscle strength and endurance. Nield et al. (2007) [16] reported improved physical function and improved dyspnea in 40 patients with chronic obstructive pulmonary disease after a 12-week pursed-lip breathing intervention, whereas Izadi-avanji and Adib-Hajbaghery (2011) [17] reported an improvement in pulmonary and respiratory function and quality of life.

Spinal joint mobilization and respiratory muscle endurance training are crucial for increasing diaphragm thickness and improving respiratory function in patients with COVID-19. Because no such study has been performed, we examined the effects of spinal joint mobilization and respiratory muscle endurance training on diaphragm thickness and respiratory function in patients previously diagnosed with COVID-19.

2. Materials and Methods

2.1. Participants

Among subjects who had been diagnosed with COVID-19 for one month, this study was conducted on subjects who met the selection criteria. The study included 30 volunteers who were recruited through an advertisement at Hospital B, a general hospital located in Gyeonggi-do. The inclusion criteria were as follows: (1) history of COVID-19 at least 1 month prior; (2) forced vital capacity (FVC) <80% of the predicted normal value and not receiving specific treatment; (3) no cardiovascular disease or depression; (4) a score of at least 24 points on the Mini-Mental State Examination—Korean (MMSE-K) and the ability to communicate and follow instructions; and (5) the provision of voluntary written consent before study participation. The exclusion criteria were as follows: (1) congenital or acquired thoracic cage deformities; (2) a history of undergoing chest or abdominal surgery; (3) the inability to perform respiratory mechanisms; and (4) orthopedic diseases of the trunk.

The study was conducted from November to December 2021 and included 30 volunteers, who were divided into thoracic mobilization and respiratory muscle endurance training (TMRT, $n = 15$) and lower limb ergometer (LE, $n = 15$) groups according to the experimental objective. To minimize selection bias, the groups were divided based on random assignment using a computer. The training program was conducted for 30 min 3 times a week for 8 weeks. Assessments were conducted before and eight weeks after the experiment. Pre- and post-test, rehabilitative imaging ultrasound was used to measure changes in diaphragm thickness. In addition, a diagnostic spirometer was used to measure respiratory function in terms of FVC, forced expiratory volume in 1 s (FEV1), and maximum expiratory rate. The study adhered to the Helsinki Declaration principles and was approved by the Gimcheon University Institutional Review Board (No: GU-202104-HRa-05-02; 21 June 2021).

The sample size determination was founded on data collected from a pilot study. We calculated the sample size using G*Power 3.1.9.7 software (Heinrich-Heine-University Düsseldorf, version 3.1.9.7, Düsseldorf, Germany). The effect size variable was right-side diaphragm contraction. The input parameters were group 1 (mean: 0.03, SD: 0.01) and group 2 (mean: 0.02, SD: 0.01). Thus, a total of 30 study subjects were calculated, (15 in each group); the effect size D was 1.2649111, the alpha error was 0.05, and the power was 0.90.

2.2. Intervention

2.2.1. TMRT Group

Spine mobilization and respiratory muscle endurance training were conducted in this group.

Spine mobilization was conducted for 15 min using the method proposed by Maitland (2005) [18]. Joint mobilization was applied according to the level of pain and restriction of movement: Grade I—low-amplitude vibration at the beginning of the range of motion; Grade II—high-amplitude vibration at the midpoint of the range of motion; Grade III—high-amplitude vibration at the end of the range of motion; and Grade IV—low-amplitude vibration at the end of the range of motion. The volunteers were asked to lie comfortably in the prone position while the upper part of the table was lowered to allow slight bending of the spine. While standing next to the volunteer, the therapist placed their metacarpals, lateral, or tibia on the spinal processes of the volunteer's thoracic vertebrae. Subsequently, Grade II–III joint mobilization was applied by extending the arm straight so that the shoulders were directly above the spine and delivering a load through the arm to the hand [18]. Central and unilateral posteroanterior and transverse mobilization were applied to the spinal segments with reduced mobility (Figure 1).

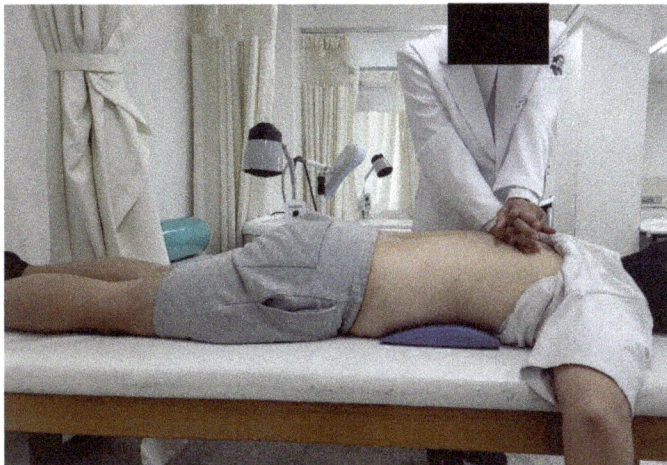

Figure 1. Thoracic spine mobilization exercise.

Respiratory muscle endurance training was conducted for 15 min. A K5 device (POWER Breathe®, Southam, UK) was used to measure the maximum inspiratory pressure while simultaneously performing the respiratory exercises. The volunteers were asked to sit with their backs straight and to inhale quickly through the mouthpiece after forcefully exhaling all the residual air from the lungs. This was repeated 30 times (one set) for three sets with a 1 min rest between sets. If the individuals complained of dizziness or fatigue, the session was resumed after a short break (Figure 2).

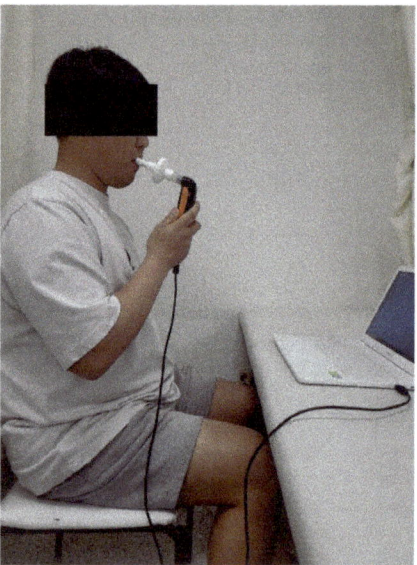

Figure 2. Respiratory muscle endurance training.

2.2.2. LE Group

The LE group performed ergometer exercises of the lower limbs. A New 3000 device (Shin Gwang, Paju, South Korea) was used for 30 min aerobic exercises. Exercise intensity was 40–50% of the maximum heart rate (HRmax) through weeks 1–4, 50–55% of the HRmax through weeks 5–8, and 55–60% of the HRmax through weeks 9–12. All individuals were asked to wear a heart rate monitor to maintain exercise intensity [19].

A pre-test was conducted before the first intervention, and a post-test was conducted after all interventions were completed. An assistant stood by for safety reasons at all times in case of a fall. A mat was prepared for the rest intervals. The devices were disinfected to prevent infection once the measurements were completed.

2.3. Evaluation

2.3.1. Diaphragm Thickness

A Rehabilitative Ultrasound Image (RUSI) digital image analyzer was used to measure diaphragm thickness. A MYSONO U5 (Samsung Medicine, Seoul, South Korea) real-time ultrasound imaging device was used for image collection. All tests used a 7.5 MHz linear transducer, 6–8.5 MHz frequency modulation, and a 20–80-grain range. The individuals were first asked to comfortably lie down, and the space between the 8th and 9th intercostal muscles along the right axillary line was marked. Subsequently, while in the supine position, the transducer was moved perpendicular to the chest wall to measure the space between the 8th and 9th intercostal muscles in a two-dimensional coronal plane. The individuals were asked to repeat the maximum inhalation and exhalation process three times to accurately measure the diaphragm thickness at maximum exhalation (at rest) and maximum inhalation (at contraction). The changes in thickness were measured, and the mean of the three measurements was calculated.

2.3.2. Respiratory Function

A PC-based spirometer (MicroQuark, Cosmed, Italy) was used to measure pulmonary function. First, the volunteers were asked to sit comfortably on a bed and hold a personal mouthpiece between their teeth with their lips covering it to prevent exhalation through the nose. The measurement variables included FVC, FEV1, and peak expiratory flow rate (PEF) after measuring maximal expiratory effort using a spirogram. The mouthpiece was immediately separated and disinfected with alcohol for hygiene purposes after each measurement.

2.4. Data Analysis

PASW for Windows (version 20.0; IBM-SPSS, Seoul, Republic of Korea) was used for all statistical analyses. The general characteristics and dependent variables were compared between the two groups before training using the chi-squared (gender) and independent t-tests (age, height, weight, and BMI). The Shapiro–Wilk test was used to assess normality. Independent t-tests were used to compare the differences in changes between the two groups after 8 weeks of training, while paired t-tests were used to examine the differences in training between the two groups following the intervention period. The significance level for all statistical tests was $\alpha = 0.05$.

3. Results

3.1. General Characteristics of the Research Subjects

The general characteristics of the subjects in the TMRT and LE groups were homogeneous (Table 1).

Table 1. Demographic characteristics of patients ($n = 30$).

	TMRT Group ($n = 15$)	LE Group ($n = 15$)	p-Value
Age (years)	23.13 ± 1.06	22.33 ± 1.45	0.12
Height (cm)	166.48 ± 7.99	167.73 ± 8.72	0.68
Weight (kg)	68.10 ± 14.55	69.40 ± 14.08	0.81
BMI	6.50 ± 1.43	7.10 ± 0.99	0.93
Gender (male/female)	9 (60.0%)/6 (40.0%)	8 (53.3%)/7 (46.7%)	0.71

Values are presented as means ± standard deviation. TMRT group—thoracic mobilization and respiratory muscle endurance training group; LE group—lower limb ergometer group.

3.2. Changes in Diaphragm Thickness

The left and right diaphragm thicknesses at rest differed significantly before and after the experiment in the two groups. The change in right diaphragm thickness at rest before and after the test differed significantly in the TMRT group (change value: 0.01 cm) compared to the LE group (change value: 0.01 cm). However, the change in left diaphragm thickness at rest before and after the test did not differ significantly between intervention methods (Table 2).

Table 2. Comparison of diaphragm thickness of TMRT and control groups.

Measures		TMRT Group ($n = 15$)	LE Group ($n = 15$)	t	p
Left side diaphragm rest (cm)	Pre-test	0.20 ± 0.05	0.19 ± 0.04	0.36	0.72
	Post-test	0.21 ± 0.04 [a]	0.20 ± 0.04 [a]		
	Change	0.01 ± 0.01	0.01 ± 0.01	2.033	0.05
Right side diaphragm rest (cm)	Pre-test	0.19 ± 0.05	0.19 ± 0.04	0.17	0.87
	Post-test	0.21 ± 0.05 [a]	0.20 ± 0.04 [a]		
	Change	0.01 ± 0.00	0.01 ± 0.00	1.06	0.03 *
Left side diaphragm contraction (cm)	Pre-test	0.59 ± 0.04	0.58 ± 0.03	0.42	0.68
	Post-test	0.63 ± 0.04 [a]	0.61 ± 0.03 [a]		
	Change	0.04 ± 0.01	0.03 ± 0.00	4.68	0.00 *
Right side diaphragm contraction (cm)	Pre-test	0.59 ± 0.03	0.59 ± 0.03	0.17	0.86
	Post-test	0.64 ± 0.04 [a]	0.61 ± 0.03 [a]		
	Change	0.05 ± 0.02	0.03 ± 0.04	5.78	0.00 *

Values are presented as means ± standard deviation; * $p < 0.05$; [a] Significant differences between pre- and post-test ($p < 0.05$). TMRT group—thoracic mobilization and respiratory muscle endurance training group; LE group—lower limb ergometer group.

The left and right diaphragm thickness during contraction differed significantly before and after the experiment in both groups. The change in left and right diaphragm thickness differed significantly in the TMRT group (change values: 0.04 cm and 0.05 cm) compared to the LE group (change values: 0.03 cm and 0.03 cm) (Table 2). The left and right diaphragm thicknesses at rest differed significantly before and after the experiment in the two groups. However, the change in left and right diaphragm thickness at rest before and after the test did not differ significantly between intervention methods (Table 2).

The left and right diaphragm thickness during contraction differed significantly before and after the experiment in both groups. The change in left and right diaphragm thickness differed significantly in the TMRT group (change values: 0.04 cm and 0.05 cm) compared to the LE group (change values: 0.03 cm and 0.03 cm) (Table 2).

3.3. Change in Respiratory Function

FVC, FEV1, and PEF differed significantly in the two groups before and after the experiment (Table 3). Regarding the change in FVC, the TMRT group (change value: 0.25 L) showed a significant difference compared to the LE group (change value: 0.09 L). Regarding the change in FEV1, the TMRT group (change value: 0.34 L) showed a significant difference compared to the LE group (change value: 0.16 L). Finally, the TMRT group (change value: 0.31 L) showed a significantly different change in PEF compared to the LE group (change value: 0.17 L) (Table 3).

Table 3. Comparison of respiratory function of TMRT and control groups.

Measures		TMRT Group (n = 15)	LE Group (n = 15)	t	p
Force vital capacity (L)	Pre-test	4.10 ± 0.44	4.09 ± 0.44	0.06	0.95
	Post-test	4.35 ± 0.36 [a]	4.18 ± 0.42 [a]		
	Change	0.25 ± 0.19	0.09 ± 0.08	3.15	0.00 *
Forced expiratory volume in the one second (L)	Pre-test	4.00 ± 0.44	3.96 ± 0.22	0.30	0.77
	Post-test	4.34 ± 0.31 [a]	4.13 ± 0.26 [a]		
	Change	0.34 ± 0.19	0.16 ± 0.17	2.72	0.00 *
Peak expiratory flow (L)	Pre-test	4.71 ± 0.90	4.62 ± 0.58	0.34	0.74
	Post-test	5.02 ± 0.76 [a]	4.78 ± 0.47 [a]		
	Change	0.31 ± 0.20	0.17 ± 0.15	2.20	0.00 *

Values are presented as means ± standard deviation; * $p < 0.05$; [a] Significant differences between pre- and post-test ($p < 0.05$). TMRT group—thoracic mobilization and respiratory muscle endurance training group; LE group—lower limb ergometer group.

4. Discussion

This study divided patients who experienced COVID-19 into TMRT (15 volunteers) and LE (15 volunteers) groups to examine their diaphragm thickness and respiratory function. The results showed significantly greater differences in the TMRT group than in the LE group.

Long-term sequelae of COVID-19 (also known as post-COVID condition, long-term COVID, long COVID, and chronic COVID) are defined as the persistence of symptoms and signs for at least 12 weeks after COVID-19 that are not explained by other diagnoses. However, there remains no global consensus on the definition; furthermore, newly emerging late-onset sequelae and changes in symptoms or conditions are also referred to as long-term sequelae of COVID-19 [20]. Among these sequelae, dyspnea reportedly occurs in one-quarter of patients following COVID-19 [21]. During a 2-month observation period, persistent dyspnea occurred in about half of patients following COVID-19, with one-third showing persistent cough and only 27% showing improvement in chest radiographs [22]. These results suggest that patients with COVID-19 require interventions for respiratory function improvement.

Thoracic mobilization increases the following: facet joint sliding of the thoracic vertebrae, thoracic flexibility by inducing chest expansion by normalizing the joint capsule, thoracic movement during inhalation, and thoracic expansion. Additionally, thoracic mobilization also helps improve lung function [23,24]. Therefore, herein, we examined the effects of TMRT and LE on diaphragm thickness and respiratory function in patients who had been diagnosed with COVID-19.

The results of this study showed significant changes in pre- and post-intervention diaphragm thickness in the TMRT and LE groups; however, no statistically significant differences were identified between the groups. This finding was consistent with that reported by Kim et al. (2013) [19] on improved diaphragm thickness in patients with stroke following breathing retraining. Kaneko et al. (2010) [25] reported that changes in diaphragm thickness were closely related to pulmonary capacity during maximum inhalation. Thus, the increased diaphragm thickness in the present study may have improved exercise performance by positively affecting the inspiratory muscles involved in physical performance [26]. The change in diaphragm thickness observed in this study may have had a positive effect through the increase in thoracic vertebrae mobility and diaphragm contraction alteration; the respiratory muscle endurance training provided active respiratory exercises.

Forced vital capacity (FVC), forced expiratory volume in one second (FEV1), and peak expiratory flow (PEF) are used as indicators to estimate levels of respiratory function [27]. The results of the present study showed significant changes in respiratory function in the TMRT and LE groups, as well as significant differences between the groups. These findings are consistent with those of a prospective cohort study by Gloeckl et al. [28], which reported improvements in 6 min walking distance, FVT, and FEV1 following respiratory rehabilitation in patients with severe COVID-19. Our study findings are also consistent with those of Liu et al. (2020) [29], who reported significant improvements in respiratory function indicators, such as FVC and FEV, and 6 min walking distance in the intervention group (where a threshold-resistant expiratory muscle strengthening device was incorporated with coughing exercises, stretching, and diaphragm training in older adults with COVID-19) compared to the control group. In addition, Mueller et al. [30] showed similar findings to a study in which the ratio of forced expiratory volume for 1 s-to-forced vital capacity and forced expiratory volume for 1 s significantly increased after a breathing exercise in spinal cord injury patients. The thoracic vertebrae mobilization exercises in this study induced thoracic vertebrae and rib cage movement, while the respiratory muscle endurance training strengthened the diaphragm, increasing the inflow and outflow of air, thereby resulting in respiratory function changes.

The limitations of this study include the following: (1) the effects of participant-dependent variables could not be completely ruled out due to the environmental factors in their daily lives; (2) the interpretation and generalization of the study results for diaphragm thickness and respiratory function changes in patients with COVID-19 are limited, as these individuals were selected based on inclusion and exclusion criteria; (3) there was no control group, so there was a lack of access to data on improvement in respiratory function over time; and (4) we did not consider the possibility that the small sample and BMI values might have confounded the results. Additional research is needed to evaluate the mobilization of various parts involved in respiratory function, different methods of respiratory muscle endurance training, and various dependent variable assessment tools.

5. Conclusions

This study's findings indicate that TMRT can be considered a potential method to improve diaphragm thickness and respiratory function in patients with COVID-19. Diversified TMRT will need to be developed for broader application of the combined approach as a therapeutic intervention for the functional recovery of patients with long-term COVID-19.

Funding: This research received no external funding.

Institutional Review Board Statement: The study adhered to the Helsinki Declaration principles and was approved by the Gimcheon University Institutional Review Board (No: GU-202104-HRa-05-02; 21 June 2021).

Informed Consent Statement: Informed consent was obtained from all subjects involved in the study.

Data Availability Statement: Data is unavailable due to privacy or ethical restrictions.

Conflicts of Interest: The authors declare no conflict of interest.

References

1. Cascella, M.; Rajnik, M.; Aleem, A.; Dulebohn, S.; DiNapoli, R. *Features, Evaluation, and Treatment of Coronavirus (COVID-19)*; StatPearls Publishing: Treasure Island, FL, USA, 2023.
2. Giuseppe, P.; Alessandro, S.; Chiara, P.; Federica, B.; Romualdo, D.B.; Fabio, C.; Simone, S.; Felice, E.A. COVID-19 diagnosis and management: A comprehensive review. *J. Intern. Med.* **2020**, *288*, 192–206.
3. Esakandari, H.; Nabi-Afjadi, M.; Fakkari-Afjadi, J.; Farahmandian, N.; Miresmaeili, S.M.; Bahreini, E. A comprehensive review of COVID-19 characteristics. *Biol. Proced. Online* **2020**, *22*, 1–10. [CrossRef] [PubMed]
4. Frownfelter, D.; Stevens, K.; Massery, M.; Bernardoni, G. Do abdominal cutouts in thoracolumbosacral orthoses increase pulmonary function? *Clin. Orthop. Relat. Res.* **2014**, *472*, 720–726. [CrossRef]
5. Hanrahan, S.; Van Lunen, B.L.; Tamburello, M.; Walker, M.L. The Short-term effects of joint mobilizations on acute mechanical low back dysfunction in collegiate athletes. *J. Athl. Train. Natl. Athl. Train. Assoc.* **2005**, *40*, 88–93.
6. Reiman, M.P.; Matheson, J.W. Restricted hip mobility: Clinical suggestions for self-mobilization and muscle re-education. *Int. J. Sport. Phys. Ther.* **2013**, *8*, 729.
7. Watchie, J. *Cardiovascular and Pulmonary Physical Therapy: A Clinical Manual*, 2nd ed.; Elsevier Health Sciences: St. Louis, MO, USA, 2010.
8. Magee, D.J. *Orthopedic Physical Assessment*, 6th ed.; Elsevier: St. Louis, MO, USA, 2014; Volume 11, p. 286.
9. Kim, K.H.; Kim, D.H. Effects of maitland thoracic joint mobilization and lumbar stabilization exercise on diaphragm thickness and respiratory function in patients with a history of COVID-19. *Int. J. Environ. Res. Public Health* **2022**, *19*, 17044. [CrossRef] [PubMed]
10. Manzano, R.M.; Carvalho, C.R.; Saraiva-Romanholo, B.M.; Vieira, J.E. Chest physiotherapy during immediate postoperative period among patients undergoing upper abdominal surgery: Randomized clinical trial. *São Paulo Med. J.* **2008**, *126*, 269–273. [CrossRef]
11. Thomas, J.A.; McIntosh, J.M. Are incentive spirometry, intermittent positive pressure breathing, and deep breathing exercises effective in the prevention of postoperative pulmonary complications after upper abdominal surgery? A systematic overview and meta-analysis. *Phys. Ther.* **1994**, *74*, 3–10. [CrossRef]
12. Moodie, L.; Reeve, J.; Elkins, M. Inspiratory muscle training increases inspiratory muscle strength in patients weaning from mechanical ventilation: A systematic review. *J. Physiother.* **2011**, *57*, 213–221. [CrossRef]
13. Dall'Ago, P.; Chiappa, G.R.; Guths, H.; Stein, R.; Ribeiro, J.P. Inspiratory muscle training in patients with heart failure and inspiratory muscle weakness. *J. Am. Coll. Cardiol.* **2006**, *47*, 757–763. [CrossRef]
14. Xiao, Y.; Luo, M.; Wang, J. Inspiratory muscle training for the recovery of function after stroke. *Cochrane Libary* **2012**, *5*, 1–27. [CrossRef]
15. Tout, R.; Tayara, L.; Halimi, M. The effects of respiratory muscle training on improvement of the internal and external thoraco-pulmonary respiratory mechanism in COPD patients. *Ann. Phys. Rehabil. Med.* **2013**, *56*, 193–211. [CrossRef]
16. Nield, M.A.; Soo Hoo, G.W.; Roper, J.M. Efficacy of pursed-lips breathing: A breathing pattern retraining strategy for dyspnea reduction. *J. Cardiopulm. Rehabil. Prev.* **2007**, *27*, 237–244. [CrossRef] [PubMed]
17. Izadi-avanji, F.S.; Adib-Hajbaghery, M. Effects of pursed lip breathing on ventilation and activities of daily living in patients with COPD. *Res. Artic.* **2011**, *2*, 1690–2046.
18. Maitland, G.; Hengeveld, E.; Banks, K.; English, K. *Maitland's Vertebral Manipulation*; Churchill Livingston: Edinburgh, UK, 2005.
19. Kim, K.T.; Cho, J.H. Effects of elastic band and aerobic exercise on fitness, blood lipids, and vascular inflammatory markers in elderly women. *Off. J. Korean Acad. Kinesiol.* **2013**, *15*, 129–138.
20. Kim, Y.J. COVID-19 and long-term sequelae. *Korean J. Med.* **2022**, *97*, 23–27. [CrossRef]
21. Sandra, L.L.; Talia, W.O.; Carol, P.; Rosalinda, S.; Paulina, A.R.; Angelica, C. More than 50 long-term effects of COVID-19: A systematic review and meta-analysis. *Sci. Rep.* **2021**, *11*, 16144.
22. Mandal, S.; Barnett, J.; Brill, S.E.; Brown, J.S.; Denneny, E.K.; Hare, S.S.; Heightman, M.; Hillman, T.E.; Jacob, J.; Jarvis, H.C.; et al. 'Long-COVID': A cross-sectional study of persisting symptoms, biomarker and imaging abnormalities following hospitalisation for COVID-19. *Thorax* **2021**, *76*, 396–398. [CrossRef]
23. Khedr, E.M.; El Shinawy, O.; Khedr, T.; Aziz Ali, Y.A.; Awad, E.M. Assessment of corticodiaphragmatic pathway and pulmonary function in acute ischemic stroke patients. *Eur. J. Neurol.* **2000**, *7*, 509–516. [CrossRef]
24. Ogiwara, S.; Ogura, K. Antero-posterior excursion of the hemithorax in hemiplegia. *J. Phys. Ther. Sci.* **2001**, *13*, 11–15. [CrossRef]

25. Kaneko, H.; Otsuka, M.; Kawashima, Y.; Sato, H. The effect of upper chest wall restriction on diaphragmatic function. *J. Phys. Ther. Sci.* **2010**, *22*, 375–380. [CrossRef]
26. Enright, S.J.; Unnithan, V.B.; Heward, C.; Withnall, L.; Davies, D.H. Effect of high-intensity inspiratory muscle training on lung volumes, diaphragm thickness, and exercise capacity in subjects who are healthy. *Phys. Ther.* **2006**, *86*, 345–354. [CrossRef] [PubMed]
27. Kisner, C.; Colby, L.A.; Borstad, J. *Therapeutic Exercise: Foundations and Techniques*; Fa Davis: Philadelphia, PA, USA, 2017.
28. Gloeckl, R.; Leitl, D.; Jarosch, I.; Schneeberger, T.; Nell, C.; Stenzel, N.; Vogelmeier, C.F.; Kenn, K.; Koczulla, A.R. Benefits of pulmonary rehabilitation in COVID-19: A prospective observational cohort study. *ERJ Open Res.* **2021**, *7*. [CrossRef] [PubMed]
29. Liu, K.; Zhang, W.; Yang, Y.; Zhang, J.; Li, Y.; Chen, Y. Respiratory rehabilitation in elderly patients with COVID-19: A randomized controlled study. *Complement. Ther. Clin. Pract.* **2020**, *39*, 101166. [CrossRef] [PubMed]
30. Mueller, G.; de Groot, S.; van der Woude, L.; Hopman, M.T.E. Time-courses of lung function and respiratory muscle pressure generating capacity after spinal cord injury: A prospective cohort study. *J. Rehabil. Med.* **2008**, *40*, 269–276. [CrossRef]

Disclaimer/Publisher's Note: The statements, opinions and data contained in all publications are solely those of the individual author(s) and contributor(s) and not of MDPI and/or the editor(s). MDPI and/or the editor(s) disclaim responsibility for any injury to people or property resulting from any ideas, methods, instructions or products referred to in the content.

MDPI
St. Alban-Anlage 66
4052 Basel
Switzerland
Tel. +41 61 683 77 34
Fax +41 61 302 89 18
www.mdpi.com

Medicina Editorial Office
E-mail: medicina@mdpi.com
www.mdpi.com/journal/medicina

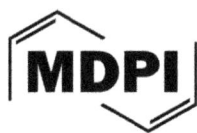

www.ingramcontent.com/pod-product-compliance
Lightning Source LLC
LaVergne TN
LVHW070042120526
838202LV00101B/412